the green cure

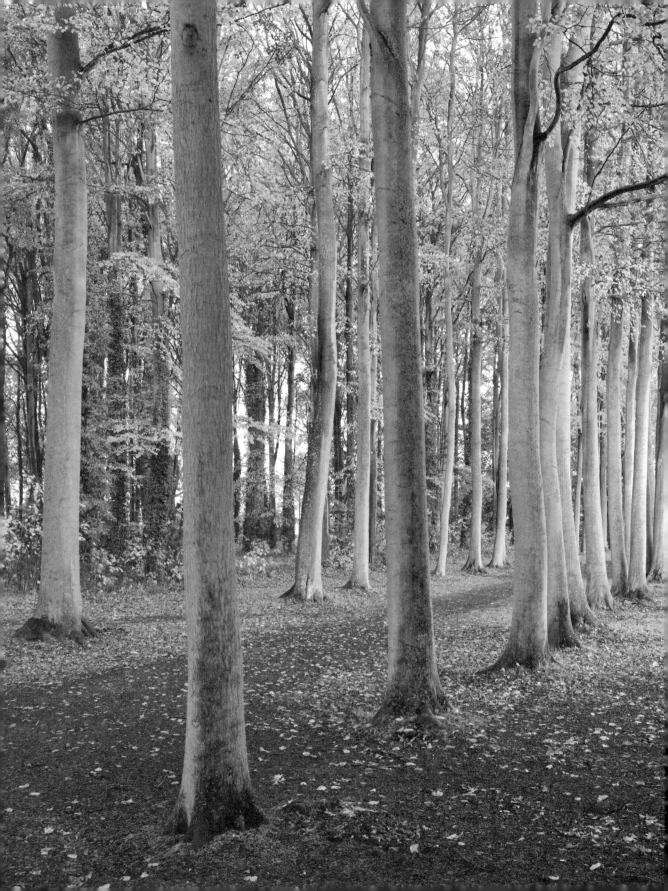

the green cure

how shinrin-yoku, earthing, going outside,
or simply opening a window can heal us

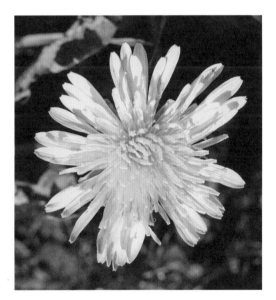

alice peck

CICO BOOKS
LONDON NEW YORK

For Duane and Tyl, always...

Published in 2019 by CICO Books
An imprint of Ryland Peters & Small Ltd
20–21 Jockey's Fields   341 E 116th St
London WC1R 4BW   New York, NY 10029

www.rylandpeters.com

10 9 8 7 6 5 4 3 2 1

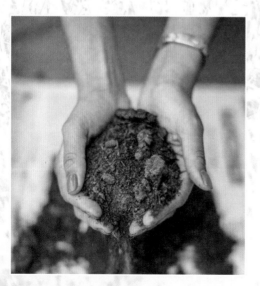

A CIP catalog record for this book is available
from the Library of Congress and the British Library.

ISBN: 978-1-78249-695-3

Printed in China

Editor: Rosie Fairhead
Designer: Emily Breen
Illustrator: Jenny McCabe

Commissioning editor: Kristine Pidkameny
Senior editor: Carmel Edmonds
Art director: Sally Powell
Head of production: Patricia Harrington
Publishing manager: Penny Craig
Publisher: Cindy Richards

Disclaimer

The information in this book including but not
limited to text and images is for informational
purposes only. It is not intended to be a substitute
for professional medical advice, diagnosis, or
treatment. The reader should regularly consult a
physician in matters relating to his/her health and
particularly with respect to any symptoms that may
require diagnosis or medical attention.

Note

Every effort has been made to contact and
acknowledge copyright holders of all material
included in this book. The publisher and author
apologise for any errors or omissions that may
remain and ask that these omissions be brought
to their attention so that they may be corrected in
further editions.

CONTENTS

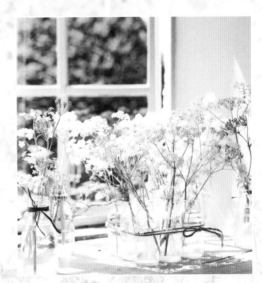

INTRODUCTION:
FROM EDEN TO ECOTHERAPY

I'm optimistic by nature, and seldom morbid, but when I'm feeling low, one of my favorite places to wander is Green-Wood Cemetery in Brooklyn, New York. It is glorious and green and quiet—very quiet. When roaming its 478 acres (193 hectares) in the middle of the most populated city in the United States, I've seen warblers and water lilies, gathered acorns and my thoughts. The verdure, the serenity, and the frogsong all bring me back to life.

I am by no means the first person to have this regenerative experience. Regardless of who we are or where we live, what we all know intuitively—and have done since paradise was envisioned as a garden—is that going outside is good for us. I call this *the green cure*: connecting to the natural world so that we can thrive physically, cognitively, emotionally, and even spiritually. In 1973, the social psychologist and philosopher Erich Fromm coined the term "biophilia," "the love for humanity and nature, and independence and freedom."[1] Just over a decade later, the biologist E.O. Wilson expanded on the idea with his own biophilia hypothesis, explaining that humans are designed with "the urge to affiliate with other forms of life," including trees, streams, and flowers.[2] In his own way, each pointed to a path to wellness and wellbeing that costs nothing and needs no equipment: the green cure.

A foundation of current science and neuroscience underlies the health-giving benefits of being outdoors. Day after day, as I was working on this book, I'd come across new and interesting reports and discoveries. Just as Western doctors and psychologists are now prescribing traditional Eastern practices such as meditation and yoga, they are also recommending that people spend time outside to remedy all sorts of ailments. According to the distinguished physician G. Richard Olds, few healing procedures work as both prevention and therapy, but being in nature is a notable exception.[3]

This current scientific understanding is proving what humans have known for millennia. Almost every mythology describes an archetypal natural realm without sickness or death, be it the biblical Garden of Eden, the Sumerian utopia of Dilmun, or the heavenly Hindu Nandankanan. Temples of Asclepius, the ancient Greek god of healing—perhaps the first sanatoriums—were built in the countryside far from centers of population. The twelfth-century mystic and saint Hildegard of Bingen, who is considered the originator of the study of natural history in Germany, often wrote of *viriditas*—usually translated as "greenness"—describing the divine healing power of green, of nature. The transcendentalists of nineteenth-century America reached the same conclusion, among them Ralph Waldo Emerson, who famously proclaimed in his essay *Nature* (1836): "I feel that nothing can befall me in life ... which nature cannot repair."

Yet, the idea of the green cure is not the exclusive domain of philosophers, mystics, and poets. There have been many manifestations of the concept—from Chinese medicine to native American healing practices—but in some ways, the green cure was most clearly articulated by Dr. Roger Ulrich, an environmental psychologist. His article "View Through a Window May Influence Recovery from Surgery," published in *Science* in 1984, indeed opened the window for modern scientists to understand how nature can heal us. He sparked much of the thinking that led to this book, and explored the science that underlies it.

Understanding and applying the idea of the green cure is a matter of taking what the medical sociologist Aaron Antonovsky termed a *salutogenic*

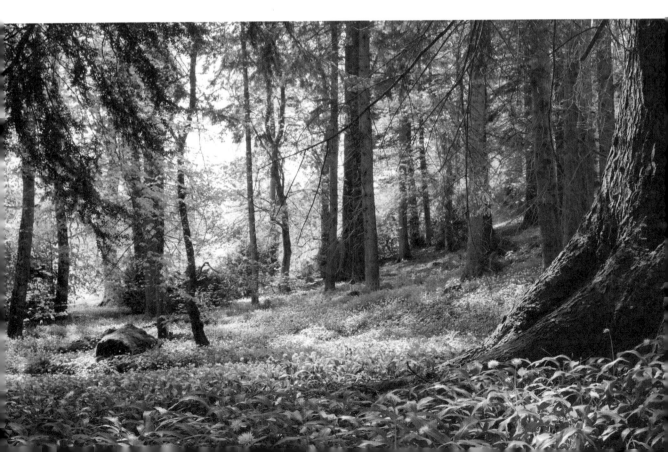

approach—involving the origins (Greek: *genesis*) of health (*salus*)—the preventative converse of the pathogenic model of seeking out the disease. Instead of focusing on the causes of disease and lack of wellness, we cultivate actions and environments that support health and wellness, which help us to thrive. Antonovsky wrote: "Life for even the fortunate among us is full of conflict and stressors, but there are many breathing spells."[4]

Thinking about those curative breathing spells brings me to meditation and neuroscience. Although I love to read about neuroscience, my understanding of it is amateur at best, and boils down to this often-quoted line from the American psychologist and writer Dr. Rick Hanson: "The brain takes its shape from what the mind rests upon."[5] That's why I've included several meditations in this book, and why I see them as a key part of the green cure. With such twentieth-century breakthroughs in technology as functional magnetic resonance imaging (fMRI), meditation and contemplation left the temple, the pew, and the ashram and entered the laboratory for observation. Researchers are now able to take pictures of the brain to discover how our neural circuits work. There is mounting scientific evidence that contemplative practices can heal us psychologically (from diminishing stress to boosting creativity), physiologically (from increasing immunity to improving heart function), and even on a cellular level.[6] As we'll see in the following pages, meditation, particularly mindfulness meditation in natural environments, can be especially restorative.

Burgeoning new fields such as ecopsychology (the study of the connection between human beings and the natural world) and ecotherapy (nature-based health treatment programs) are gaining acceptance among physicians and psychologists. Some of these practitioners call themselves "bioneers," looking to nature to remedy the ills of our bodies, our communities, and the planet. Like me, they believe nature can help to heal our bodies, our minds, and even our spirits. Often, it's just common sense, something as simple as taking a moment to pause, notice, and breathe. Vacation days aren't a requirement; we can connect with nature even when we're very far from the countryside or seashore and can't leave our home or workplace to be outside. There are myriad ways, both large and small, to seek out nature in our day-to-day lives. It may be a view from a window or a potted plant on a desk, but the green cure is almost always available and free for the taking.

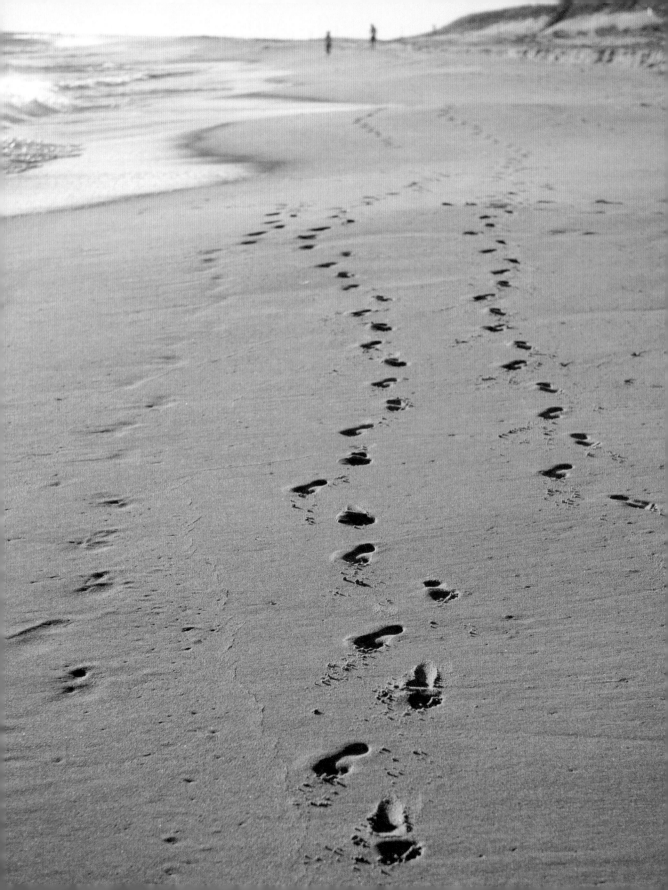

CHAPTER 1

FRESH AIR

*Doth not the air breathe health, which
the birds, delightful both to ear and eye,
do daily solemnize with sweet consent
of their voices?*

Sir Philip Sidney,
The Countess of Pembroke's Arcadia (1590)

THE WONDERS OF
AN OPEN WINDOW

As I was writing this book, friends often asked me what it was all about. I may have waxed enthusiastic about the thrill of new scientific discoveries concerning health and nature, about how so many things we had always intuited about wellness could now be empirically proven, especially through breakthroughs in neuroscience, and about the undeniable connection between psyche and body. Then, I would explain that the entire book can be encompassed in one sentence: *Open a window and you will feel better.* It's true. Try it right now. Stand up, walk over to the nearest window, and open it. If you are in an office building or a rainstorm (or both) and can't open a window, at least sit by one. Take a deep breath. Look up into the sky or let your gaze settle on something green—a tree, a hedge, a flower bed, a potted plant. Take another breath.

Did you notice a shift? I'm guessing you did. Chances are you slowed your heart rate, drew in a little more (probably cleaner) oxygen, which improved your focus and concentration, and gave your back a bit of a stretch. You gathered your thoughts and, even for the briefest of moments, felt part of the world beyond yourself—mindful and connected. Your mood may have improved. All this in less than a minute, and without a gadget, supplement, or special clothing or shoes! If that's not wonderful, I don't know what is.

The idea of opening a window to make us feel better is not new. As one Miss Mollet wrote in *A Noble Profession: Nursing the Sick* in 1887, "Cleanliness and ventilation are one and the same thing." Dr. Roger S. Ulrich, Ph.D. EDAC, was a trailblazer in evidence-based healthcare design—the scientific relationship between a built environment and the impact it has on the people who use it—and appears quite a bit throughout this book. Ulrich was the first to gather and publish data on how merely looking through a window can help to heal us. He examined patients recovering from gallbladder removal surgery in a hospital in Pennsylvania between 1972 and 1981. Of the 200 patients he studied, 23 were assigned to rooms looking out on deciduous trees, while the others had a view of a brick wall. He published his results in an article, "View through a Window May Influence Recovery from Surgery":

Twenty-three surgical patients assigned to rooms with windows looking out on a natural scene had shorter postoperative hospital stays, received fewer negative evaluative comments in nurses' notes, and took fewer potent analgesics than 23 matched patients in similar rooms with windows facing a brick building wall.[1]

Remarkable! All from looking at a few oaks, maples, or elms. As far as I can tell, Ulrich's study was the first formal one on this subject, but it has been supported by many since. One done with pulmonary patients in 2011 showed that by measuring mental health, subjective wellbeing, and emotional states, as well as other markers, "an unobstructed bedroom view to natural surroundings appears to have better supported improvement in self-reported physical and mental health."[2]

- This research has gone beyond hospitals: University students who had natural views scored better in tests than those who did not;

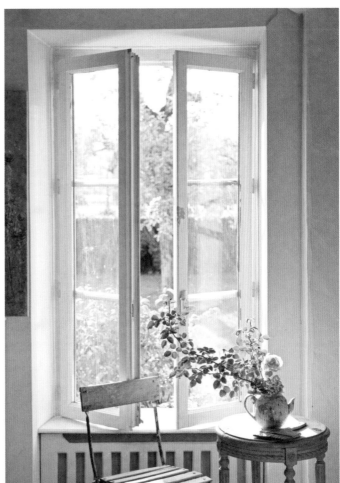

- Prisoners who saw greenery through their cell windows suffered fewer stress symptoms, digestive illnesses, and headaches, and made fewer visits to the doctor;

- Office workers with a view of trees and greenery described their jobs as less stressful and were more satisfied with their occupations than those who had a view limited to other buildings;

- Likewise, those employees with a view of nature considered quitting their jobs less frequently.[3]

The positive effects of seeing nature can occur pretty much anywhere. A researcher at the University of British Columbia, Holli-Anne Passmore, recently studied the connection between taking a moment to look at something from the natural environment and personal wellbeing. For two weeks, 395 participants were instructed to write down how the nature they encountered during their daily routine—a houseplant, a dandelion growing in a crack in a sidewalk, birds, or sun through a window—made them feel, and take photos of the things that sparked those feelings. Other participants did the same with human-made objects, and a third group did neither.

According to Passmore, "This wasn't about spending hours outdoors or going for long walks in the wilderness ... this is about the tree at a bus stop in

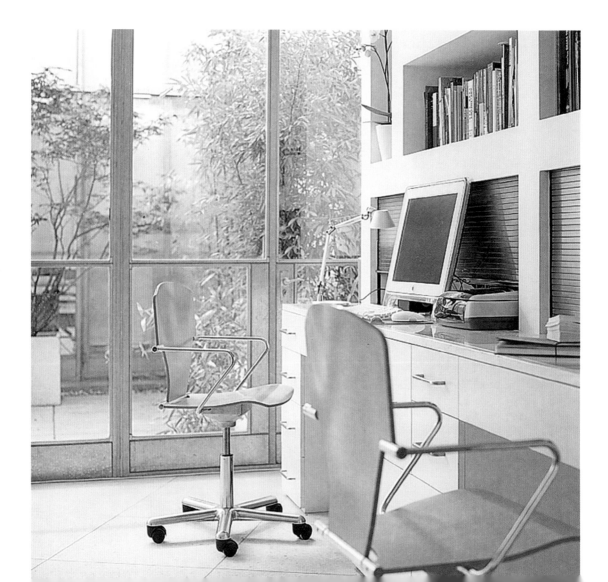

the middle of a city and the positive effect that one tree can have on people."[4] She was "overwhelmed" not only by the positive responses but also by observing how much more joyful the "nature group" participants seemed, and how they expressed a sense of connection to nature *and* to other people, than the group that focused solely on human-made objects. So it follows that taking pictures of the sunrise or roses as they're about to bloom can not only delight you but also improve your relationship with the people around you.

It's what comes through the window as well

The green cure can be found not just in what we see through the window, but also in what comes in. Even if the weather is cold, pulling back the curtains or opening the blinds and giving yourself a break from artificial light can improve your state of mind. There is a genuine connection between how much daylight we are exposed to and how well we sleep. The neuroscientist Ivy Cheung, while doing post-doctoral work at Harvard Medical School's Division of Sleep Medicine, found that the amount of daylight that workers are exposed to has a remarkable impact, and for the sake of the wellness of employees we should consider how our office buildings (or any workplace) incorporate natural light.[5] This is because artificial light doesn't balance our circadian rhythms—our sleeping/waking cycles over a period of twenty-four hours—the way natural light does, and of course it doesn't apply solely to the workplace. (I'll explore this further in Chapter 9.)

Looking out of a window and receiving light through it are both valuable, easy actions to take to improve our physical, psychological, and maybe even spiritual wellbeing, but the benefits multiply when we open those windows. Take vitamin D, for example. The human need for it has been well established, and a deficiency can lead to all sorts of medical problems such as malabsorption of nutrients and rickets, a softening of the bones. One of the best ways to get vitamin D is through exposure to sunlight, since the sun emits ultraviolet waves that set off a chemical reaction when they reach the skin, creating vitamin D. But the important thing is that although sunshine can pass through glass, the ultraviolet waves cannot, so if you want to increase your intake of vitamin D, sit by an *open* window.

Beyond vitamins

There is more to an open window than vitamin absorption. When you were a child and your mom told you to go outside and get some fresh air, she was onto something. That's why the World Health Organization recommends fresh-air ventilation as a way to diminish the transmission of communicable diseases, such as tuberculosis. Interviewed in *Scientific American*, the infection control specialist Rod Escombe of Imperial College London described a study he had carried out in Lima, Peru, in which he compared the airflow of seventy rooms in eight hospitals that treated tuberculosis patients. If windows and doors allowed air to flow, the air in a room was fully replaced about twenty-eight times per hour—even more than if ventilation fans were used without open windows (only about twelve times per hour). Escombe recommended that waiting rooms have access to the outdoors, that hospitals have larger windows as well as skylights that can open, and that tuberculosis wards be downwind of other areas.[6]

Think about this in terms of your everyday life—perhaps not tuberculosis, but the common cold. You've probably noticed that you tend to get sick more often after spending time in an enclosed space with lots of people, such as in the cabin of an airplane, a classroom, or the doctor's waiting room. When air can't circulate, the odds of germs cycling and recycling through our systems increase exponentially. Bill Sothern, an expert in indoor air quality and the founder of Microecologies, told the *New York Times*: "The air indoors is 10 times more contaminated than the air outdoors at any given time."[7] This can lead to headaches, asthma, allergies, lethargy, and dermatological conditions in homes, schools, workplaces, hospitals, and anywhere else that people congregate.

So open that window, and do your best not to close it when you go to bed. We rest more deeply and for longer not just if we're exposed to natural light during the day, but also if there is a constant flow of fresh air during the night. A study published in the journal *Indoor Air* found that in ventilated spaces where the air circulates there is less carbon dioxide buildup. Although it is crucial for many things (including photosynthesis of plants), carbon dioxide is the gas that we exhale, flushing impurities from our bodies. Lower carbon dioxide levels in the air around us lead to deeper, longer, and less interrupted sleep.[8] Our bodies don't have to work so hard to do their jobs of cleansing our cells, lungs, and blood, and so we can better settle and rest.

Or take it a step farther. Try taking your bed outside. Victorian houses were built with sleeping porches, and homes in the Middle East and India have courtyards that allow fresh air to circulate, improving the quality of their residents' rest and likely diminishing instances of disease by diffusing germs. Perhaps you have a porch or balcony that you can set up for sleeping during clement weather? Or, if you live in an apartment building, maybe you could "camp" on the roof on a summer night?

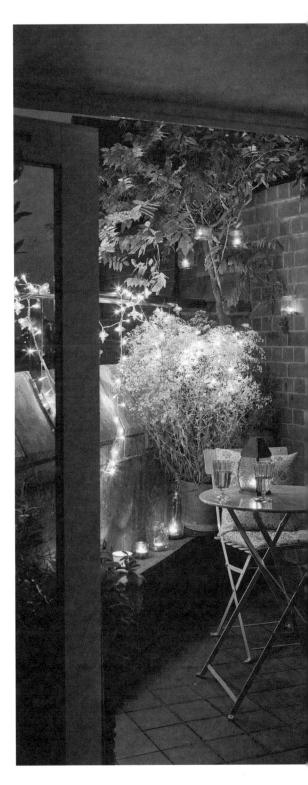

The air outdoors

Sometimes a real camping trip is a possibility. It's one of the least expensive ways of taking a vacation, and has many of the greatest benefits. Camping has become more popular recently, perhaps in part because it allows us to escape from our digital lifestyles. Hashtags such as #vanlife and #optoutside have gone beyond trends to become phenomena, arriving at the everyday.

However, camping is more than a craze or a backdrop for ad campaigns to sell bottled water. Some researchers consider it the best treatment for TILT (toxicant-induced loss of tolerance), a condition wherein our immune system sustains too much exposure to toxins, whether human-made pollutants such as pesticides and cleaning agents, or natural ones such as smoke, pollen, or dust mites. It is no small thing: A life without enough fresh air can lead to numerous physical and mental ailments, including chronic pain and abnormal brain activity.[9]

(I just got up, opened my front door, and took some big, deep breaths. What about you?)

Camping—which allows us to get large doses of clean air over a prolonged period—may be a way to dilute or clear out the toxins in our systems, but we must be aware of this every day, even when a vacation is not an option. This kind of understanding helps to illuminate why *friluftsliv* is such an important element of Scandinavian culture. The term, which means "open-air living" or "free air life," was coined by the nineteenth-century Norwegian writer Henrik Ibsen in his poem "On the Heights," which is in part about the benefits of solitary retreat:

> In the lonely mountain farm,
> My abundant catch I take.
> There is a hearth, and table,
> And *friluftsliv* for my thoughts.[10]

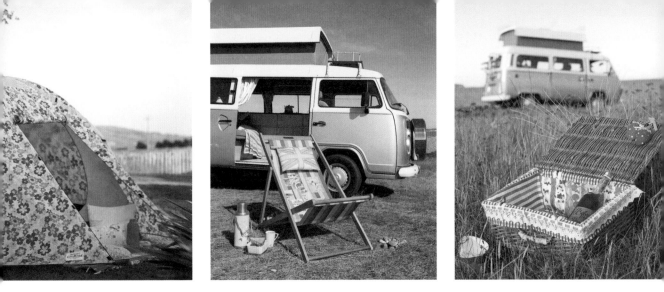

There is a possibility that for Ibsen, *friluftsliv* was a way to mitigate his chronic depression and anxiety. Data that compares the health of Scandinavian cultures, for whom *friluftsliv* and a connection to nature is a way of life, with that of countries or populations that neglect to spend time outdoors regularly supports this.

The benefits of fresh air go beyond easing depression. According to the Natural Resources Institute Finland and others, there is a correlation between lowered stress and a few moments of connection with green space.[11] Again, even gazing out a window will do the trick. If we take it a step farther and spend five hours in nature outside an urban environment, preferably in two or three "doses," our mood and state of mind will improve markedly.[12] Five hours per month—less than ninety minutes a week—spending time in a park, the woods, or a garden seems quite manageable for most of us.

Fostering connection

There is a deeper element to looking out a window. When we do so, we get out of our own heads and connect with the world beyond the self. It's not an insignificant thing. Sometimes we have no time to engage with other people, but it can be healing to know that they are there. Looking out of a window in the city and seeing your fellow humans can create a sense of connection, commonality, and compassion: Perhaps they are going through a difficult time ... they found love ... they survived childhood ... they're tired after a long day at work—just like us.

Observing nature can foster a similar feeling of interconnection. It can make our problems feel smaller and give us context within the vastness of the universe, a sense of peace and awe. When I think of the times I have felt most spiritually connected, they have not been dramatic or calculated—at retreats or organized events—but in small moments of perception: the whisper of a breeze through the trees, a startlingly blue sky, raindrops splattering on an iron bannister, the sudden appearance of ducklings out of tall grass.

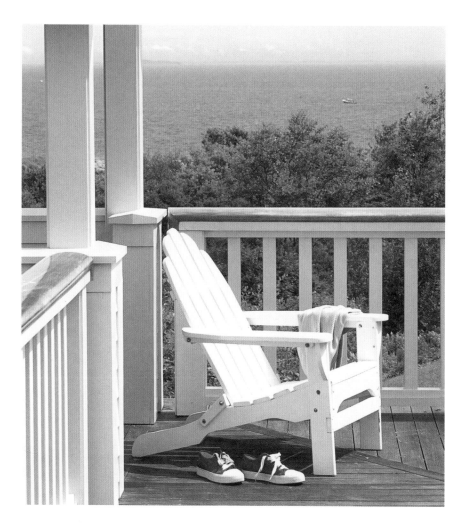

WINDOW TIME

There are thousands of self-help books with prescriptions both basic and labyrinthine to help us live, think, and feel better, but here is one of the simplest and yet most reliable suggestions you are likely ever to find: *Pause and look out the window.* This tiny action can change your mood, your day, your way of being.

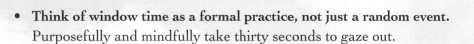

- **You may find it helpful to create a reminder for yourself.** I set the alarm on my phone, but you might prefer to connect the action mentally to specific points in the day, such as after you have eaten a meal or as soon as you arrive at work or school.

- **Think of window time as a formal practice, not just a random event.** Purposefully and mindfully take thirty seconds to gaze out.

- **It can be a kitchen window or a train window,** looking onto a forest or a single sapling, no matter—with active intention and attention, do that one thing: Look out the window.

- **Try it for a few days and pay attention to any changes** in the moment and later in the day. Do you notice a positive result?

If you like window time, you'll love what comes next!

CHAPTER 2

TAKE A WALK

Above all, do not lose your desire to walk: every day, I walk myself into a state of well-being and walk away from every illness; I have walked myself into my best thoughts, and I know of no thought so burdensome that one cannot walk away from it.

Søren Kierkegaard (1813–1855),
from a letter to his sister-in-law Henriette

AGE MORE SLOWLY, LOVE MORE, AND SPARK CREATIVITY

Opening a window is good, but going out into nature is even better. It is normal to feel refreshed by a walk outside; it's a way to dust the cobwebs from your mind, welcome a new perspective on the day or on life, and get the blood flowing. Taking a walk is all about getting a change of scene and, ideally, encountering a little green.

Any kind of walking is good for you, but outdoors is best. You will get even more vitamin D—the sunshine vitamin—from that than from sitting near an open window. You will also experience a better physical and mental workout navigating uneven outdoor terrain rather than the consistent surface of a treadmill. And there's a bonus! It is hard to be on a smartphone or other device when you are walking outside, so you will also give yourself a break from screens. There are many other benefits to going for a walk. You will be able

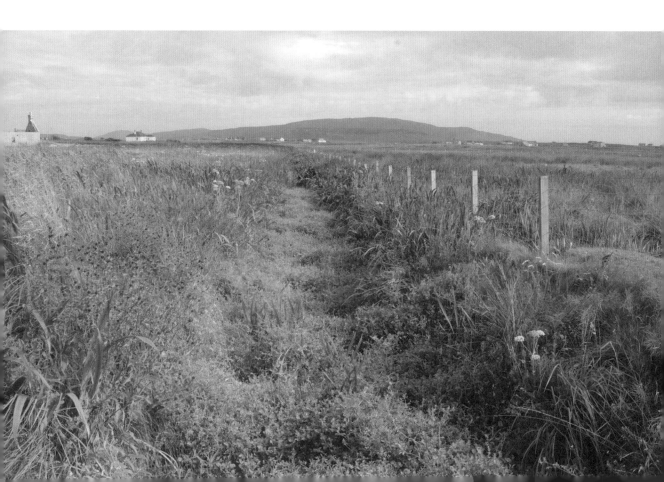

to greet and maybe get to know other walkers, thereby connecting with people and building community, and you can do your own small part for the environment by picking up a bit of trash to improve the aesthetics of your route.

Chairs are the new cigarettes

Healthcare practitioners are saying that chairs are the new cigarettes. *Seriously*—too much sitting can kill you! Or, as Kierkegaard put it, "the more one sits still, the closer one comes to feeling ill."[1]

Research from the University of California found that sitting for too long—like smoking—increases the risk of diabetes, heart disease, and even early death. The researchers found a connection between sedentary behavior and thinning in parts of the brain that are responsible for forming memories.[2] This can be a precursor to dementia and other types of cognitive decline, and middle-aged and older adults should be especially aware of it.

A famous comprehensive study published in the *Journal of Clinical Nutrition* analyzing 240,000 Americans between the ages of 50 and 71 showed a direct correlation between sitting and mortality.[3] The more we sit, the sooner we die. It sounds dire indeed, but the good news is that the converse is also true: By getting up and moving we delay the onset of many age-related problems.

For example, the effect of aerobic and ambulatory exercise on Alzheimer's disease was studied by scientists at the University of Kansas. Half the test subjects engaged in walking and brisk movement, while the other half did toning and stretching exercises. All showed some improvement in tests for physical skills, but what is fascinating is that "some of the walkers significantly increased their scores on cognitive tests that focused on thinking and remembering. The brain's hippocampus, the area most closely linked to memory retrieval, had in some cases actually grown."[4] Think about that: We can develop our brains by taking regular walks.

That's just the beginning. Walking also helps with:

- The reduction of inflammation, osteoporosis, and cardiovascular disease;
- Enhanced balance, posture, and joint fluidity, and even a lowered incidence of vascular dementia;
- Improved digestive health and a colon that functions better;
- "Good" cholesterol levels, and lowers triglycerides or "bad" cholesterol.[5]

It has an especially significant impact on the vagus, the nerve that connects our brain to our body, branching out to our primary organs (heart, lungs, and digestive tract). It's the nerve that makes the mind/body connection. When you activate the vagus nerve by walking, yoga, deep breathing, steady stretching, or any kind of rhythmic exercise, it regulates your adrenal gland, which produces hormones in stressful situations, and modulates blood pressure and the flow of blood to the organs, especially the heart, allowing them to function more efficiently and effectively.[6]

Happier in motion

It's not just in our bodies that we see the benefits of fresh air and movement; with physical fitness comes psychological fitness. Poets, painters, scientists, and efficiency experts have all commented on how outdoor exercise in nature works as a balm for our minds and a way to de-stress. How many times have you taken a walk around the block to cool off? Or sent a whiny child outside to play?

Former competitive racewalker and cancer survivor Carolyn Scott Kortge supports this idea in her book *Healing Walks for Hard Times: Quiet Your Mind, Strengthen Your Body, and Get Your Life Back* (2010). She reveals how taking a walk is about far more than exercise; it can serve as "a form of stress release and healing that supports medical treatment and emotional recovery." The basic ambulatory act increases our exhalations and inhalations, causing us to release endorphins—from the term "endogenous morphine"—that trigger a natural opioid effect, making us feel happier and more optimistic, while decreasing our perception of pain. It's those hormones that cause the well-known "runner's high."

Numerous studies have shown that walking encourages the front region of our brain—the hypothalamus, which controls temperature, thirst, and hunger, and affects sleep and emotions—to manufacture oxytocin, often known as the love hormone. This acts as a neurotransmitter in the brain, stimulating feelings of empathy and affection. And with love often comes happiness. Walking can make us more joyful. A series of studies by the University of Michigan showed that this was true no matter one's age—from schoolchildren to the elderly.[7]

These benefits to our health have to do with overriding rumination—our tendency to dwell on troubling thoughts or worry about everything from finances to our child's hurt feelings. These are the kinds of thought tinged with sorrow that we can't seem to let go of. Long-term rumination, marked by activity in the part of the brain that controls emotions and the personality (the prefrontal cortex), can lead to depression.

Walking in nature has been shown to decrease rumination. A Stanford University study found that taking a ninety-minute walk through a natural environment as opposed to an urban one reduces rumination and consequently the neural activity in the part of the brain that is linked to the risk of mental illness.[8] Findings such as these reinforce why green spaces are so crucial for good mental health, especially for those of us who live in urban areas.

When it comes to happiness, *how* you walk matters. According to the *Journal of Behavior Therapy and Experimental Psychiatry*, people who were instructed to walk in a happier manner, with a lively, energetic gait, experienced more positive thoughts (as indicated by biofeedback

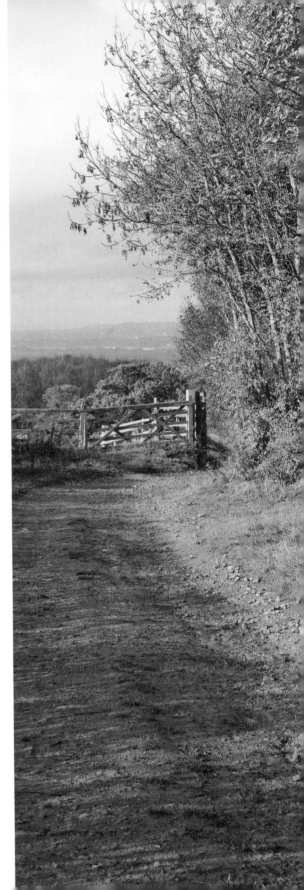

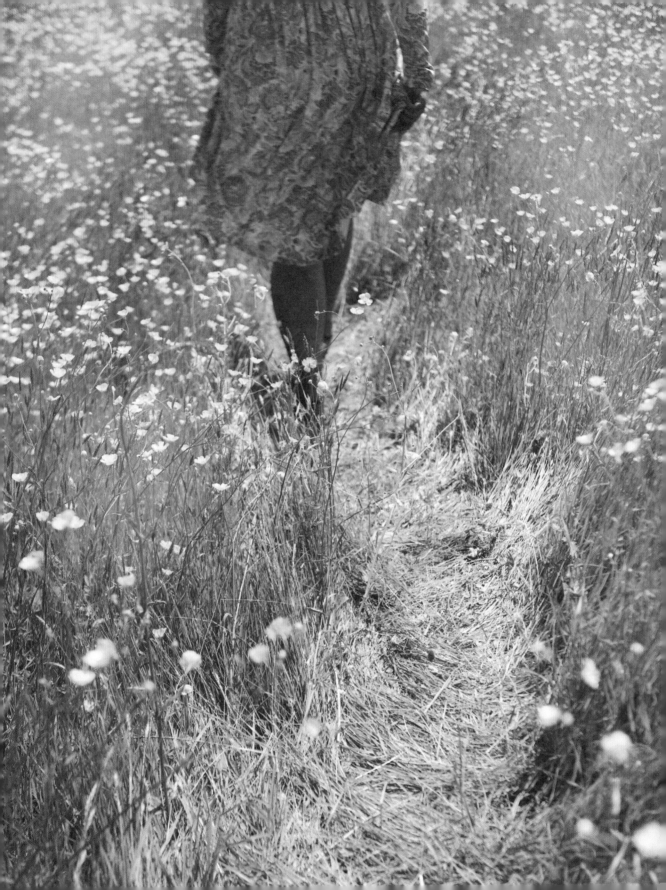

testing, which monitors indicators like heart and breathing rate and blood pressure), recalled them more readily, and had fewer depressive tendencies.[9] It is like the expression "acting as if": If you act as if you feel better, you begin to feel (at least a little) better. A simplified explanation is the adage "the neurons that fire together, wire together." By thinking happier thoughts, we become happier thinkers.

Myriad articles and studies detail the cognitive benefits of interacting with nature, in part because it captures our attention subtly ("Is that a bluebird?"), as opposed to walking in an urban environment ("Watch out for that car!"). This was quantified by researchers from the University of Michigan, who examined memory tests of students after sending them for a brief walk in an arboretum. They showed a 20% improvement in memory after interacting with nature, even in wintry weather, so it was the outdoors and not specifically the greenery that seemed to help.[10]

A study presented in the *Proceedings of the National Academy of Sciences* in 2015 supported this. Its researchers found that walking in a park reduced blood flow to a part of the brain that causes rumination, thereby improving positive focus.[11] I like to ponder, and perhaps dwell, and sometimes that can get overwhelming, so this study struck a chord for me.

150 minutes per week

The great thing about reaping the benefits of walking is that we don't have to do very much to change our health for the better. In most of the research I read (and which you can find details of at the end of this book), 150 seems to be the magic number: People who engaged in 150 minutes of walking per week showed marked improvements and benefits. So, if you can, make moving for at least 25 minutes six times a week your goal. Think about walking the dog or strolling to the market, getting off the subway or bus a stop before your destination, taking the scenic route home, running up and down the stairs in your apartment building on rainy days. All these things can change your life significantly.

Of course, the more you walk, the better, but experts say that while it's good to aim for a whole lot of steps, your focus should be on sustaining consistent daily minimums, not sporadically pushing yourself to reach a record number of steps. A sports tracking device or smartphone app could come in handy with this. It will help you to keep track of time and see how quickly 25 minutes can pass when you're both in motion and in nature.

Rambles, treks, and wanderings

In his essay "The Etiquette of Freedom" in *The Practice of the Wild* (1990), the poet and ecologist Gary Snyder describes walking as "the great adventure, the first meditation, a practice of heartiness and soul primary to humankind ... the exact balance of spirit and humility." Recent Harvard University studies on green space and health confirm what he said: that walking heals more than our bodies and minds, but also our spirits, even our creative spirits.

Writers from Henry David Thoreau to Rebecca Solnit, and from Jean-Jacques Rousseau to Jane Austen, have pointed out the link between walking and creativity. Two researchers at Stanford University, Marily Oppezzo and Daniel Schwartz, analyzed this theory and found that walking—whether outdoors or indoors—enhanced creativity, especially when brainstorming new ideas. It didn't matter whether the subjects walked on a treadmill facing a bare wall or out in nature; test results showed that participants who walked before being asked to find creative solutions to problems performed twice as well as those who remained sedentary.[12]

Walking outdoors can be especially good for the spirit, which is perhaps why people have always been drawn to pilgrimages such as the Camino de Santiago (popularized during the Middle Ages as a route of Christian pilgrimage, the paths through northwest Spain are still a favorite among hikers of all faiths) or the trail to the Shinto shrine at the top of the Nachi Falls in Wakayama Prefecture, southern Japan. This is a way of embodying the sacred journey, as our inner, mental voyage is reflected and marked by an outer, physical one.

A trudge through a vacant lot can be as beneficial as a stroll through a meadow, if it's all that is available. Whether it is a pilgrimage or a trip around the block, try to find time each day to engage with the world around you, being present and appreciating the simple beauties of nature. Try taking off your headphones, or—and this is really hard for me, because I like a purpose, whether it is a trip to the market or exercising the dog—try ambling, walking without a purpose or destination in mind.

There are many reasons to recommend the writer and former Zen Buddhist monk Clark Strand's beautiful meditation on sleep, dark, and light, *Waking Up to the Dark* (2015). He writes about how our nightly patterns break into three parts when we are removed from artificial light for a significant amount of time: about four hours of deep sleep, two hours of awakened quiet rest, then four more hours of sleep. We'll go into the reasons for this, and other matters of light and dark, in Chapter 9, but meanwhile one of my favorite things about Strand's book is his descriptions of walking at night: "If someone asked me why I rise to walk at night, I couldn't answer except to say that I do it for its own sake, for the sake of rising and walking and praying in the dark. That time of contemplation and communion is its own reward. It creates its own culture in the soul."[13]

Ever since I read Strand's treatise about the things we can see without artificial light, I've been taking little walks in the dark—not the mountain hikes he describes, but around my house or into the backyard in darkness. It's a kind of meditation: By removing visual distractions we can become more present, more mindful of where we are.

WALKING MEDITATION

The Vietnamese Buddhist teacher and peace activist Thich Nhat Hanh wrote in *Present Moment, Wonderful Moment* (1990):

> The mind can go in a thousand directions.
> But on this beautiful path, I walk in peace.
> With each step, a gentle wind blows.
> With each step, a flower blooms.[14]

Like exercise, the benefits of meditation are many, and scientists and doctors are always finding new ones, from easing stress to improving focus to facilitating healing on all levels from heart health to immunity. There is a way to combine both exercise and meditation, and you can do it outside in nature, whether that nature is a sylvan glade, a seashore path, or the sidewalk between apartment

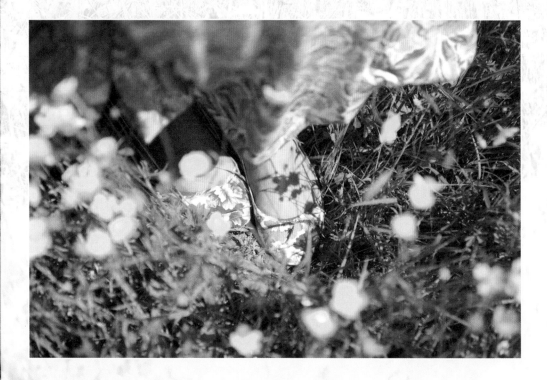

buildings. Here is a walking meditation practice based on the Zen technique *kinhin*, which might seem familiar if you have ever intentionally walked a labyrinth. It can be done inside or outdoors, but try for as much fresh air and greenery as possible. It's best if you plan your route in advance. Knowing your destination means you won't have to make decisions and can pay attention to each step:

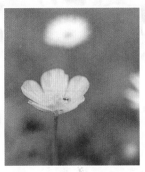

- **Stand up straight** and take a deep breath.

- **Hold your hands in such a way that they don't swing** around but won't cramp either. I like to fold mine in front of me, the left held in the right.

- **Synchronize your breath with your pace.** Inhale and step slowly and deliberately, exhale and take another step.

- **Begin to walk, paying attention to lifting your foot and placing it on the ground,** then lifting your other foot and placing it on the ground.

- **Continue to walk in this careful, controlled manner.** Don't force it, but don't saunter either.

- **As with any mindfulness practice,** when thoughts arise, look at them and let them go. Don't ignore, don't judge.

As you walk, consider repeating this simple nature mantra, often recommended by Thich Nhat Hanh when he teaches:

*"Breathing in, I know Mother Earth is in me.
Breathing out, I know Mother Earth is in me."*

CHAPTER 3

SHINRIN-YOKU

In the woods, we return to reason and faith. There I feel that nothing can befall me in life—no disgrace, no calamity ... which nature cannot repair. Standing on the bare ground, my head bathed by the blithe air, and uplifted into infinite space ... the currents of the Universal Being circulate through me.

Ralph Waldo Emerson, *Nature* (1836)

THE PROVEN HEALTH BENEFITS OF TIME WITH TREES

Any walk outdoors is good for you, but if you can get to some woods, that's even better. Over the past few years, more people have become intrigued by the concept of forest bathing—healing through the contemplative practice of intentionally spending time with trees—and it has really caught on. Forest bathing is being taught and practiced at botanic gardens, spas, spiritual retreats, and recreation centers. Beyond that, it is being used in psychiatric hospitals, in conjunction with physical therapy, and in addiction treatment programs.

As humans, we are drawn to trees. It's an innate tendency, and something powerful happens to us when we are near them. A love of trees transcends borders and cultures. Many people respond with delight to a mention of trees, and many will describe a special tree or a meaningful or even profound experience involving one. In his wildly popular book *Forest Bathing: How Trees*

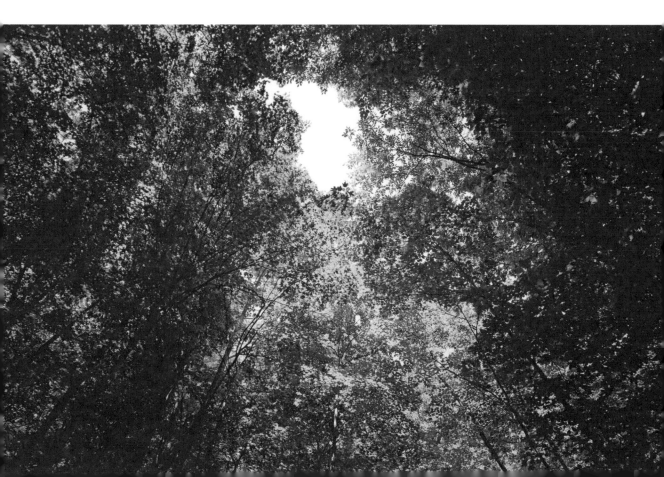

Can Help You Find Health and Happiness (2018), Dr. Qing Li explains that there is a Japanese word for that indescribable feeling: *yūgen*, meaning "deep" and "mysterious." In the Japanese system of aesthetics, it is understood as a profound and sometimes poignant wonder at the beauty of the universe. A passage by the thirteenth-century Japanese poet Kamo no Chōmei evokes this idea elegantly: "It is similar to an autumn evening under a colorless, quiet sky. Somehow, as if for a reason we cannot quite recall, tears well irrepressibly."

Yūgen is one of many reasons that forest bathing has caught on, but there are more: It is a lovely way to pass the time in nature; it is a way to connect to the spiritual without dogma; and, of course, most humans like trees. If that weren't enough, there is also a scientific explanation for how and why forest bathing makes us feel so good.

About forest bathing

In 1982, Tomohide Akiyama, then secretary of Japan's Ministry of Agriculture, Forestry, and Fisheries, coined the term *shinrin-yoku*. This translates as "forest bathing," and can be defined as making contact with and being affected—both physically and mentally—by the atmosphere of the forest. Perhaps more aptly called forest *basking*, since neither soap nor tub is involved, forest bathing can be experienced as a type of meditation, and, just as with other Eastern-rooted practices such as mindfulness, Ayurvedic medicine, and yoga, Westerners are learning that there is far more to meditation than simply becoming calm. Many authorities are in agreement that meditation can ease psychological problems from anxiety to post-traumatic stress disorder, help to treat addiction, make us better parents and workers, and promote the healing of many physical ailments.

Forest bathing incorporates many of the benefits of meditation while getting us outdoors and in motion. In a recent study conducted by the College of Landscape Architecture at Sichuan Agricultural University, Chengdu, China, thirty men and thirty women were given a route of the same length to walk in either a bamboo forest or an urban area. The results showed that, although walking is good for you, walking among trees is much better.[1] The researchers measured blood pressure as well as electrical activity in the brain using an EEG (electroencephalogram), and they found that, among those who walked the

forest path, blood pressure was lowered significantly as attention and concentration improved. The people walking in nature reported less anxiety and a generally happier mood than the urban group.

Forest bathing has an impact on even more than mood and blood pressure. The New York State Department of Environmental Conservation and myriad other sources maintain that the simple act of intentional, attentive time with trees:

- Decreases fatigue;
- Has immune-system boosting, antiviral, and even anti-carcinogenic benefits;
- Increases the ability to focus, even in children with attention-deficit hyperactivity disorder (ADHD);
- Speeds up recovery from surgery or illness;
- Regulates the endocrine (hormonal) system;
- Lowers blood glucose, affecting obesity and diabetes;
- Enhances the ability to relax and get a better night's sleep;
- Increases energy;
- Has been shown to increase brainwave activity in young adults and positively affect elderly patients with chronic heart failure.[2]

Imagine if a pharmaceutical company could produce one pill that was capable of doing all that!

Forest bathing is an active process, not just a matter of being near trees as static objects. Many species, including pine, yew, hop hornbeam, and sugi, emit biochemicals called phytoncides that interact with our central nervous system and have calming, anesthetic qualities, even anti-carcinogenic properties. Phytoncides are pungent essential oils, antimicrobial volatile organic compounds. When you are breathing in the heady fragrance of pine or cedar, you are inhaling phytoncides. They have been proven to boost the trees' health as well as our immune systems, which is a powerful thing, but that's not the only benefit of forest bathing.

Phytoncides contain terpenes (like those in cannabidiol, CBD, a chemical compound found in marijuana oil) that can stimulate immunity and anti-cancer proteins in our bodies, fight viruses, and increase the release of the steroid hormone dehydroepiandrosterone (DHEA) into the blood, protecting and even strengthening our hearts. They also activate the vagus nerve (see page 26), reduce our production of the stress hormone cortisol,[3] (making us more calm and focused), and likely decrease inflammation, as well.

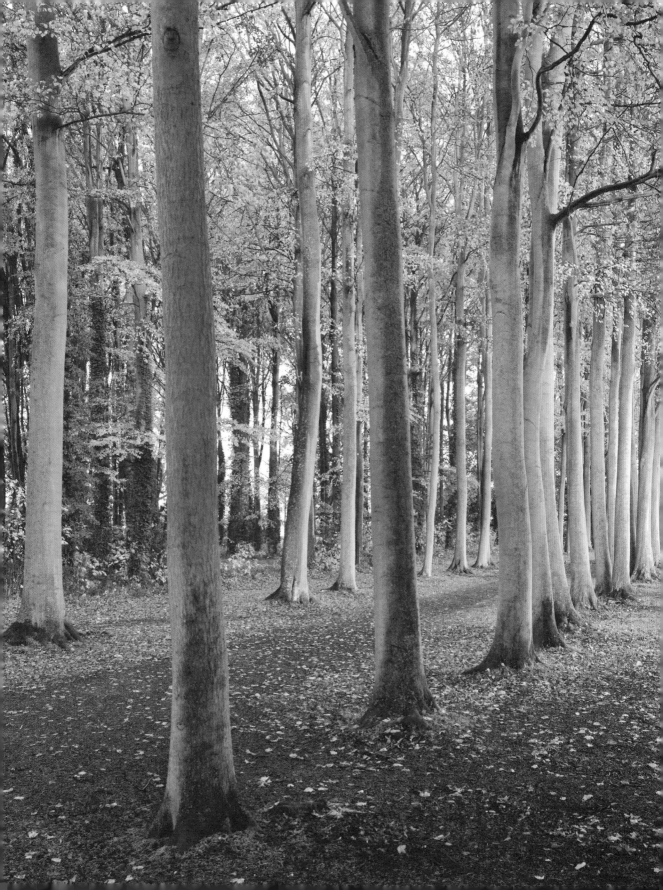

As trees emit, they also absorb. According to the German forester and writer Peter Wohlleben in *The Hidden Life of Trees* (2015), trees act as natural air purifiers, not unlike houseplants. Trees take in pollutants such as nitrogen oxide, ammonia, sulfur dioxide, and ozone through their leaves. That's part of why we feel better when we go for a walk in the woods. Breathing cleaner air is not just a pleasant experience; it can reduce the symptoms of asthma, make exercise more efficient because we don't have to work as hard to take in oxygen, and perhaps even mildly cleanse our organs.

Hearing trees

It has been scientifically proven that trees emit not just an aerosol of healing phytocides, but also beneficial sounds. We've all heard branches groan in a storm and the susurration or whispering of leaves as they move together in an afternoon breeze, but plants (and trees in particular) also emit vibrations that can be measured using microphones and ultrasonic sensors. In an interview

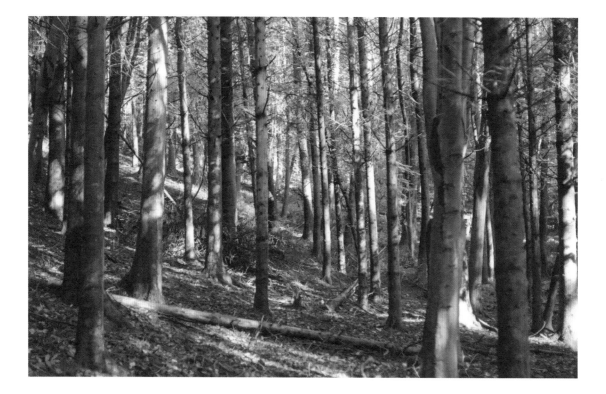

with *Yale Environment 360* in 2017, the biologist David George Haskell explained that:

> an ultrasonic detector applied to a tree, particularly in the summertime, reveals how as the morning passes into afternoon, the tree goes from a state of full hydration to a place of distress, where there are all sorts of little ultrasonic clicks and fizzles emerging from the inside of the tree as water columns break, as the tree becomes more dried out. By applying an ultrasonic sensor, the tree suddenly has its inner life revealed.[4]

Amazing!

Just as trees respond to increases and decreases in light and temperature, they also respond to sound via vibrations. For example, urban trees tend to grow thicker bark as a reaction to the shaking and pulsation of passing traffic. There are also hypotheses that trees use sounds to communicate with *one another*. In an interview in *Smithsonian* magazine, Wohlleben calls this the "wood-wide web": the connection among trees in a healthy forest, whereby nutrients and water are shared and information sent by means of a symbiotic relationship underground, between microscopic filaments at the tips of tree roots and fungi—called mycorrhizal networks—to signal threats such as drought or insect infestation.[5]

If trees can emit vibrations, it follows that human beings can pick them up, even if only on a very subtle level. Maybe there is something to tree-hugging after all? I spoke to several proponents of forest bathing who say that it is those vibrations that can cure headaches more quickly and naturally than taking an analgesic. I haven't had that experience, but I do know that when my thoughts are unsettled, if I sit with the silver maple in my backyard I feel better. Is it the vibrations, the terpenes, the green of the leaves, or the pause to reflect on something that has endured more than a hundred years of blizzards, thunderstorms, and heatwaves? I'm not sure, but I know it heals me in a unique way.

City trees

We can't all get to the woods, but fortunately, as we've already seen, there are health benefits to even a little bit of nature. A park, a tree-lined road, or a couple of trees in a backyard or courtyard can help.

Urban planners and environmental scientists are taking the benefits of forest bathing to heart and working to create more effective green spaces. One initiative is City Tree, which isn't a tree at all, but rather a structure built from mosses that bind with toxins and particulates to clean the air.[6] It looks a bit like a giant television, but instead of a flat screen, a huge patch of moss covers the vertical surface. Not only does the moss clean the air, but also, because it stores a considerable amount of moisture, it cools the area around it.

Projects to plant (real) city trees are cropping up all over the world as urban planners learn more and more about the power of green. The MillionTreesNYC initiative was launched by the New York City Parks Department in 2007, and the project's goal was achieved in 2015. A million street trees were planted throughout the city over a period of eight years. As part of the scheme, the non-

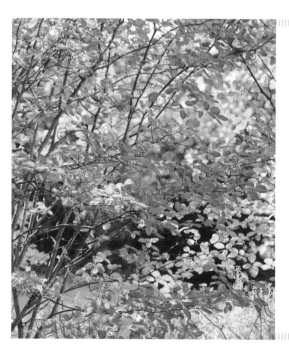

Finding the right trees

It is important to note that not all forests are rich in phytoncides. Wohlleben points out that when spruce and pine trees are introduced to places where they're not indigenous, the trees suffer, dry out, and create excess dust, making us less, not more, healthy, so be aware when seeking out a forest to walk in or planting trees.

profit New York Restoration Project targeted neighborhoods that needed trees, and sought out public and private funding to provide them. Other cities, including London, Shanghai, Denver, and Los Angeles, have developed similar programs, and the results are all good—from cheering up neighborhoods to raising property values to filtering air and decreasing noise pollution.

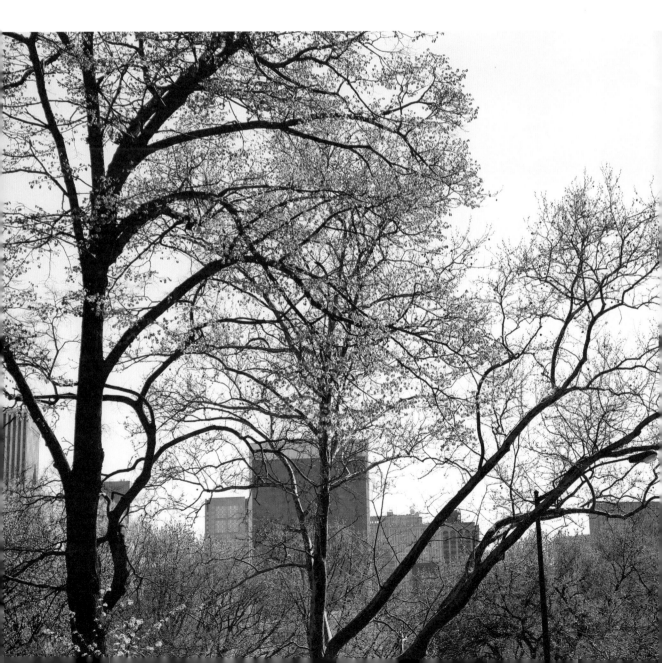

FOREST BATHING: STEP BY STEP, TREE BY TREE

So, how does one go about forest bathing?

1. **You need only the most basic equipment:** walking shoes and insect repellent. Leave your camera, your journal, and your guidebooks behind, and turn off your mobile devices. Forest bathing is about being, not analyzing.

2. **Find some trees.** This can be a forest of ancient pine or a copse of paper birch, or, if you're like me, a single silver maple in your backyard. Of course, spending more time with more trees is better, because the effect is multiplied—studies have shown that spending three days and two nights in a thickly wooded area will improve the function of the immune system for up to seven days—but do the best you can. A little forest bathing is better than none, and there are benefits to it even if you can't take in a huge lungful of phytoncides.

3. **Find somewhere to sit or lean,** where you can be still for ten or twenty minutes or more without being in the way of bicycle traffic, ants, or poison ivy.

4. **Now do just that—*be still*.** Be aware of your breath, but don't force it. Let the experience come to you, don't analyze. See what you see, hear what you hear, smell what you smell, feel what you feel. Light through the leaves … skittering or birdsong … blossom or decay … calm or grounded …

5. **As you walk home, check in with yourself.** Do you notice any changes in your body? How about your state of mind? What can you take from your forest bathing experience back to your daily life? Do you feel more optimistic? More serene? How is that headache?

6. **Repeat as often as possible,** and pay attention to any improvement in your wellbeing. Try a new spot next time, or focus on another kind of tree, and note the difference. (Having said that, forest bathing with the same trees in the same spot will vary every time, depending on the season, the weather, the time of day, and what you bring to the experience.)

Perhaps as you do this you will think about these powerful lines from Haskell's book *The Songs of Trees* (2017):

We're all—trees, humans, insects, birds, bacteria—pluralities. Life is embodied network. These living networks are not places of omnibenevolent Oneness. Instead, they are where ecological and evolutionary tensions between cooperation and conflict are negotiated and resolved. These struggles often result not in the evolution of stronger, more disconnected selves but in the dissolution of the self into relationship. Because life is network, there is no "nature" or "environment," separate and apart from humans. We are part of the community of life, composed of relationships with "others," so the human/nature duality that lives near the heart of many philosophies is, from a biological perspective, illusory.[7]

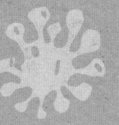

CHAPTER 4

DELIGHTFUL DIRT

May we exist in muddy water
with purity like a lotus.

Zen Buddhist chant

EARTHING, MUD BATHS, AND WELLBEING

Consider the fragrant and beautiful lotus flower—a symbol of divine perfection, especially for Hindus and Buddhists. It grows best in the mud. As the Vietnamese spiritual teacher Thich Nhat Hanh often says, "No mud, no lotus." Although our culture tends to shun dirt—and often for good reason—maybe we have gone too far. A bit of mud can be a wonderful thing. Toddlers who find joy in splashy, squishy springtime mud puddles may be onto something. Anyone who gardens knows that digging in the earth makes them feel better, and now there's science to back it up. "Good" bacteria form part of microbiomes that build our resistance to illness and fight the "bad" bacteria that cause infection. These microbiomes reside in specific environments, such as our gut, our skin, and the soil.

About the microbiome

In 2004, after learning about the successful results of using bacteria to treat drug-resistant pulmonary tuberculosis, a British oncologist injected the microorganism *Mycobacterium vaccae* (SRL172) into patients with non-small-cell lung cancer to see if it would strengthen their immune systems. It didn't work, but there was a different and surprising result: When SRL172 was combined with chemotherapy, it significantly improved the quality of the patients' lives.[1]

As indicated by their global health score (a standardized measure of respondents' evaluation of their health), those who received the injections of bacteria were happier and livelier, and had improved cognitive function.

In part because of this, three American and international research groups—the University of Chicago, the Marine Biological Laboratory, and Argonne National Laboratory—have joined together to form the Microbiome Center, a coordinated interdisciplinary research group. Its director, Jack Gilbert, explains that the microbes in our guts communicate with our brains in several ways.[2] They activate the immune system and produce neurotransmitters (chemical messengers between nerve cells), including 90% of our serotonin. This is important because serotonin contributes to happiness and wellbeing. Targeted treatments using the microbiome show promise in treating people suffering from PTSD and depression.

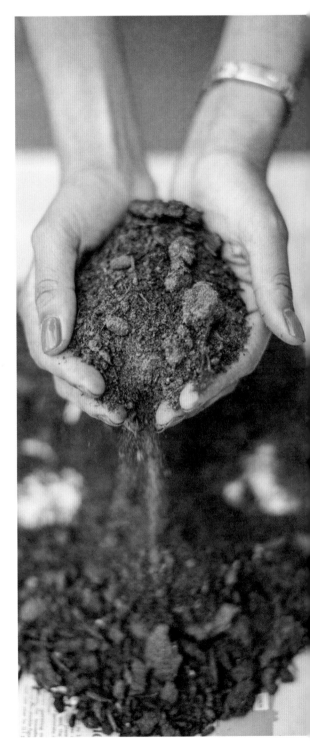

Healing mud

All this research boils down to something quite simple: Encourage your children to play in the mud! It's definitely worth the cleanup time. According to the pediatric neurologist Maya Shetreat-Klein MD, author of *The Dirt Cure* (2016), when we kill "bad" bugs—whether insects or germs—by over- or misusing pesticides, antibiotics, and hand sanitizers, we're also killing the "good" bugs that prevent ailments such as asthma, allergies, eczema, and other autoimmune problems. That's why Shetreat-Klein is often quoted as saying, "The cleaner we are, the sicker we seem to get."

How can we go about getting just the right amount of dirt? There are plenty of simple ways to meet your MDDR—Minimum Daily Dirt Requirement. Start by forgoing hand sanitizers, and consider your medicine before you take it and your food before you eat it. I think the best way to do this last is to eat organically grown fruits and vegetables as close to where they've been grown as possible. You'll certainly consume fewer pesticides, and probably a little more healthy dirt, since local, farm-grown food tends to be less sterilized and scrubbed than factory-grown. (A warning to pregnant women and anyone with a compromised immune system: wash food thoroughly to remove soil-borne toxoplasmosis.)

When it comes to small children, it may be a simple matter of encouraging them to dig in the dirt and sit on the grass, if you have access to a bit of lawn or some flowerpots. Little ones love observing bugs and small creatures, and organizing activities or adventures around such basic interests will not only get them in contact with dirt, but also give them a break from television and small screens. As children get older, encourage outdoor sports, hiking, camping, or helping in the garden. Ask your school what programs they provide to get kids outdoors—perhaps fossil-hunting for a geology curriculum or taking local soil samples for biology study.

Eat dirt?

Of course, the beneficial effects of healthy gut bacteria aren't limited to children. Eat dirt—if that's your thing! It's called geophagy, which the dictionary defines as "the practice of eating earthy substances (such as clay) that in humans is performed especially to augment a scanty or mineral-deficient diet or as part of a cultural tradition."

It's not completely crazy. Many sources explain that the reason animals and people eat soil, which is after all organic material—the stuff of plants and animals, or a salad and steak in a different form—is to ingest minerals such as iron and calcium that are necessary for our dietary health. The nutritional anthropologist Sera Young expands on this by explaining that clay works as a type of purifying filtration system, and that "it is often used to clean up massive oil spills and absorb unwanted scents from places (think kitty litter) ... it may have a similar effect in the human body, acting as a mud mask for the gut."[3]

Young isn't talking about the clay you might dig up in your backyard, but rather about the chalky clay kaolin, from the mineral kaolinite, which is common all over the world, and eaten as a folk remedy in the American South. The science is still pretty sketchy, and the process unappealing, so I'm not going to take up geophagy at this point in my life. Fortunately, there are other, more pleasant ways to contribute to a good gut microbiome and get a modest amount of dirt into our systems. One way is to eat a variety of foods, especially:

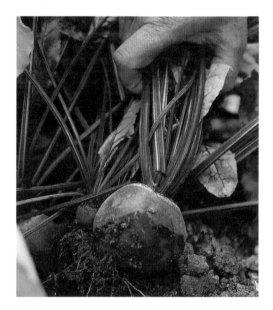

- A plant-based diet of fruits, vegetables, and legumes—stuff that grows in the dirt. Potatoes, beets, leeks, onions, and garlic are particularly suitable. (Potatoes eaten with the peel contain about twice as much potassium as bananas, and are rich in magnesium, among other nutrients.)[4]
- Fermented foods such as yogurt and kimchi, which contain *Lactobacillus*, bacteria that contribute to gut health and may even fight inflammation.[5]
- Prebiotic foods—foods that are high in fiber, such as wholegrains—that require other bacteria, such as *Bifidobacterium*, to break them down, lowering the risk of obesity, heart disease, and diabetes.[6]
- Deep-colored foods such as cocoa and blueberries that are rich in polyphenols, plant compounds that reduce blood pressure, inflammation, and cholesterol. Polyphenols aren't always absorbed efficiently or quickly by

human cells, so they must work their way down to the colon, where they can "feed" or be digested by good bacteria.[7]

Alcohol, antibiotics, smoking, and stress all have a negative impact on our gut bacteria, so limit or avoid as appropriate.

Earthing

All this shows that there's more to dirt than just, well, dirt. But it's unlikely that we'll be injecting ourselves with *Mycobacterium vaccae* or snacking from our window boxes anytime soon. As well as eating fresh fruit and vegetables, there are other ways of getting your minimum daily requirement. That's why the earthing movement is catching on. (Some say it's the next forest bathing!) Earthing involves walking barefoot and connecting directly to the soil without the barrier of pavement or shoes. It is a matter of contact with our soil, our planet, of truly touching the earth. More a question of appreciation than a scientific concept, earthing is also a way of connecting to others celebrating nature.

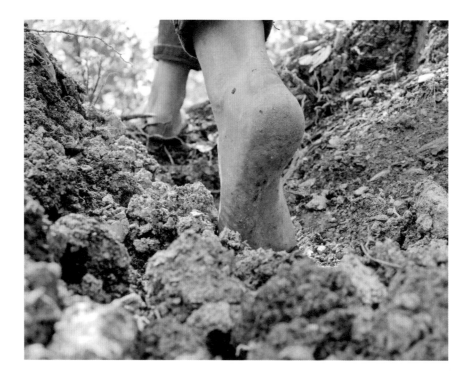

Some people take the idea a step farther, reaching beyond the biological material to the electromagnetic charge generated by our planet. The science is still fairly new and limited on this subject, but interesting nonetheless. According to the *Journal of Inflammation Research*, studies done in several disciplines have shown how grounding or earthing–the electrically conductive contact between human bodies and the Earth's surface–seems to have an effect on health. Sparking this connection between people and the ground we walk on may diminish inflammation, enhance immunity and wound healing, and prevent or even treat chronic inflammatory and autoimmune diseases. Grounding may also lessen pain by altering the numbers of circulating white blood cells (neutrophils and lymphocytes) affecting inflammation.[8] It sounds promising and will certainly bear more research.

Think of the non-scientific meaning of the word "grounded"–balanced, sensible, understanding what's important in life–and it follows that standing firmly on the earth, bonded to where we came from and where we'll end up, will have an impact.

Mud baths

If walking barefoot isn't your thing, consider fangotherapy–a mud bath! Studies have shown that applying mud to the skin can relieve psoriasis and atopic dermatitis as well as rosacea, eczema, acne, and generally itchy skin. Fangotherapy has also had proven results in treating neurological, rheumatologic (osteoarthritis), and even some cardiovascular disorders.[9] Researchers at the Kaplan Medical Center in Rehovot, Israel, found that using mudpacks and mineral-water soaks to absorb minerals through the skin may benefit our immune system. For example, sulfur baths have been successfully used to treat types of dermatitis and psoriasis, and have shown potential in regulating the skin's immune response as a treatment for allergic reactions.[10]

Where the mud comes from determines its benefits. It's those microbes again! The scientists at the Kaplan Medical Center analyzed mud from the Dead Sea, which is especially rich in organic substances such as calcium, magnesium, and potassium, and not the mud you might dredge up from the bottom of your local lake, for example. The makeup of the mud not only allows nutrients to be absorbed into the skin, but also means that it retains heat for a long time, stimulating blood flow–nature's heating pad.

CLEANSING WITH MUD

A trip to the Dead Sea or even to a spa in Calistoga, California, where a mud bath costs upward of $100, isn't a possibility for most of us. However, we can replicate some of the results at home.

1. **Make some mud.** Don't even think about dipping into your flowerpots—"clean" dirt is key. Bentonite clay or Fuller's earth (both inexpensive—about $10 per pound in the US—and available online or from health-food stores) are the best bet.

2. **Mix it with water until it reaches a workable muddy consistency,** not soupy but not powdery either. I use filtered or distilled water because to my mind it seems purer, but in truth, tap water is likely fine.

3. **Use the mud to make a face mask.** My son loves this because it really scrubs his pores. (First, test it on a small patch of skin for about 10 minutes and wait for an hour or two to make sure you don't have any sensitivities.) Simply apply a thin paste of the mud, let it soak in and dry thoroughly for about twenty minutes, wash off completely, and moisturize as much as you need to. (And don't forget to clean the sink!) You will find that your skin looks cleaner because the mud has bonded with and absorbed oils, and that it has a bit of a glow, because when you removed the mud it took dead skin cells with it.

4. **This is my favorite part: get your hands dirty!** I like to coat my hands with the mud mixture and let it dry. Like everyone, I use my hands constantly for everything from typing to cooking, and the mud soak feels therapeutic, kind of warm and toning, especially if I take the time to sit in the sun while it's drying. Once the mud has dried

Warning

Remember that because mud is all about bacteria, you shouldn't put it on an open wound or use it with infants or the immune suppressed.

fully, rinse and scrub it off. This makes my hands feel remarkably clean and look a little younger, and hopefully I've absorbed some minerals in the process.

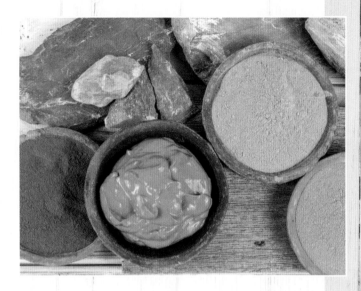

5. **Mud can be applied to injuries,** such as a sprained wrist or an arthritic knee. Although the term "mud pack" is commonly used, what is really meant is a thick mask—a heavy application of mud that is allowed to dry over the affected area. Again, heat will help, and the line between taking the time to attend to the muscle and the powers of mud itself is a blurry one.

As you're experimenting with mud, remember this verse from "Music" by the nineteenth-century American poet Ralph Waldo Emerson:

'Tis not in the high stars alone,
Nor in the cup of budding flowers,
Nor in the redbreast's mellow tone,
Nor in the bow that smiles in showers,
But in the mud and scum of things
There alway, alway something sings.

CHAPTER 5

PLANT THERAPY

*And the secret garden bloomed
and bloomed and every morning
revealed new miracles.*

Frances Hodgson Burnett,
The Secret Garden (1911)

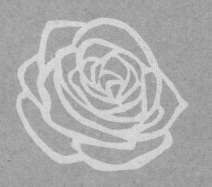

FLOURISHING IN MEADOWS, GARDENS, AND GREENSPACES

Playing with mud is fun, but my favorite way to get my Minimum Daily Dirt Requirement and connect with the earth is to dig in it. Gardens have provided a sanctuary for healing body, mind, and soul since the beginning of recorded time; some splendid examples are the imperial gardens of ancient China, the hanging gardens of Babylon, and the groves surrounding Plato's Academy and Aristotle's Lyceum. My little patch of green in Brooklyn is significantly less magnificent, but it is just as therapeutic. While digging in the earth I sort my thoughts, improve the world around me in a small yet meaningful way, and engage deeply in a few moments of active mindfulness—intentional and focused action that slows the onslaught of nagging thoughts and inner chatter.

For me, no other experience evokes and sustains what the pioneering psychologist Mihaly Csikszentmihalyi defined as "flow," a state "in which people are so involved in an activity that nothing else seems to matter; the experience is so enjoyable that people will continue to do it even at great cost, for the sheer sake of doing it."[1] It's that experience of becoming immersed in an activity, so "lost" in it that the self falls away. When I'm in the garden I rarely notice the passage of time, and all my anxieties and to-do lists evaporate. I'm not alone in this; people who love to garden will agree that it's a way to free the mind from stress-producing rumination through beauty and play, while getting a little physical exercise as a bonus.

Gardening is even better in a group. Community gardens or farms are a source of fresh seasonal and local produce, but, more importantly, they build, well, *community*. They range from allotments—land that is divided into small plots, each one leased to an individual for growing vegetables and/or flowers—to "guerrilla" gardens, where fallow or abandoned land is reclaimed and cultivated by a neighborhood for growing food and communal use. The benefits are myriad. According to Gardening Matters, an independent organization dedicated to community gardeners in Minnesota, such gardens also:

- Reduce our carbon footprint by cutting the distance that vegetables are shipped;
- Increase property values by adding green space;
- Provide employment, education, and entrepreneurship opportunities;
- Offer a supply of fresh, seasonal, nutritionally rich produce that is particularly valuable in neighborhoods that might not otherwise have access to it;
- Lower crime rates by getting people out of their homes and gathering them together in a shared enterprise;
- Provide educational and cross-cultural opportunities;
- Reduce stress and increase a sense of wellness and belonging through a shared activity, improving our state of mind.[2]

The association between gardening and the mind is not a new one. Ancient Egyptian physicians are said to have recommended walks in gardens, and during the Middle Ages monastery gardens were recommended as a place to treat melancholy. As the medieval healer and mystic Hildegard of Bingen put it, "With nature's help, humankind can set into creation all that is necessary and life sustaining."[3]

In recent years, gardening has come to be understood as a useful and effective treatment for disorders of the mind—autism, depression, and PTSD—and body, including coordination problems and rehabilitation after surgery. We have used this healing power

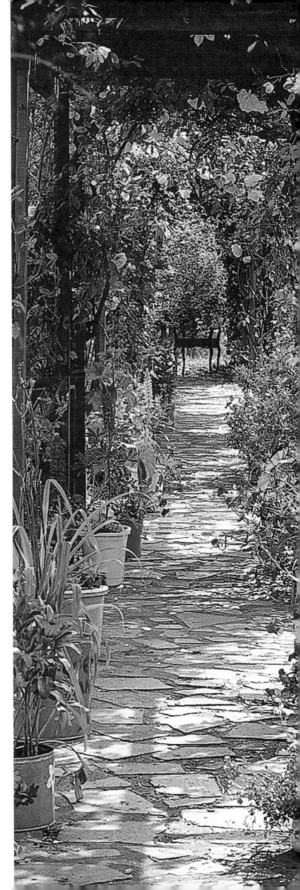

intuitively for millennia, and now studies have begun to confirm it. For example, after performing a stressful task, test subjects in a study undertaken in the Netherlands were randomly assigned half an hour of either gardening outdoors or reading indoors.[4] The researchers measured levels of cortisol (the stress hormone), and the participants kept track of their moods. It was found that both gardening and reading lowered cortisol during recovery from stress, but the decrease was significantly greater among the gardening group, who manifested better moods than the reading group. I'm sure most gardeners would agree that time spent turning compost, cutting back raspberry bushes, and tending tomatoes can provide relief from even the most acute stress. (Although that doesn't mean one should *always* opt for the garden over a good book!)

Two long-term (sixteen-year) studies of people in their sixties and seventies who gardened regularly found that the gardeners had a 36–47% lower risk of dementia than non-gardeners, even when other variables were taken into account.[5] Other studies have found that people diagnosed with depression, mood swings, or bipolar disorder who spent six hours a week tending flowers and vegetables showed a quantifiable improvement after three months.[6] What's especially interesting is that they continued to improve even after the program ended, showing that some rewiring may have occurred during the process.

Japanese researchers have found that simply looking at a garden has advantages.[7] They arranged for subjects (women whose average age was in their mid-forties) to sit in chairs and do nothing but appreciate the view of a kiwi-fruit garden for ten minutes. Compared with the control group, which had a view of buildings, the women who looked at the kiwis showed a significant increase in parasympathetic ("rest and digest," as opposed to "fight or flight") activity and a decrease in heart rate, and reported feeling more relaxed and at ease. There are many implications to all this research, but one small one is that it may be helpful to take a periodic gardening break whenever possible.

Therapeutic gardens

A practical application has sprung up from these studies: horticultural therapy. Sometimes called ecotherapy, it is any kind of green activity that has an impact on mental health. This can include the occupational therapy aspect of working in a garden and experiencing the sequence of planting, tending,

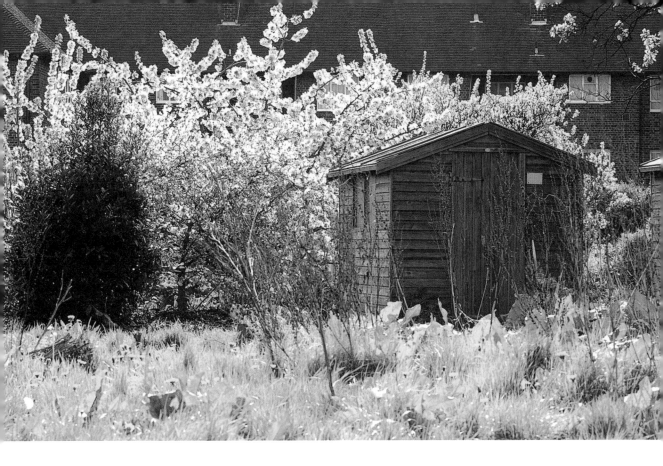

and harvesting, but it might also be a practice of integrating the senses by encountering tactility (furry pussy willows or fuzzy silver sage, for example) or fragrance. It takes place most often in a specially designed garden, but it can occur anywhere that participants interact with nature. Studies have shown that therapeutic gardens have a positive impact on memory, problem-solving, and social and language abilities.[8] The physical act of gardening can rehabilitate and strengthen muscles and restore or improve endurance, balance, and coordination. Horticultural therapy in a vocational setting teaches participants both how to work independently and how to follow directions.

School gardens

Educational gardens are also gaining popularity in schools all over the world, and their learning possibilities range from ecology and earth science to cooperation and problem-solving. In *Ripe for Change: Garden-Based Learning in Schools* (2015), Jane S. Hirschi explains that teachers tend to find that school gardens are an especially engaging learning environment for pupils. They can use the time they spend in the garden to explore several subjects—not just botany, but even areas such as geometry, when considering the structure of plants and their growth patterns, fostering multidisciplinary learning. Edible learning gardens also allow teachers to get nutrition and food education into the curriculum without diminishing the time they spend on core academic subjects: "The schoolyard garden is a sensory-rich change in environment from the classroom, and it is just outside the door."[9]

The value of gardens for children doesn't end with the school day. A recent study using MRI to gauge working memory and inattentiveness, conducted on 253 children by the Barcelona Institute for Global Health, found a correlation between the greenness of a neighborhood and the development of both white and gray brain matter, affecting both memory and attention. The report explained that this supported the "biophilia" hypothesis—that evolution has wired humans to seek out a connection with nature (see page 6)—and recommended green spaces to provide children with places for activity and rest, and opportunities for discovery, problem-solving, and learning, so as to have a positive impact on their brain development. The institute went on to report that greener areas tend to have less air and noise pollution, and that breathing healthy air containing "good" microbes could also have indirect benefits for the development of the brain.[10]

Open spaces

In her lovely book *Zen of the Plains: Experiencing Wild Western Places* (2014), Tyra A. Olstad writes an ode to "windswept ridges and wind-rent skies." She describes our tendency to dismiss wide-open spaces as empty, meaningless, and blank—devoid of the complexity of ocean or woods, for example. Setting out to understand these easily overlooked areas and to learn the power of their open-ended potential, she found meaning in the "simple sweep of the horizon; the rich color of the air." She concludes the book with "a brief meditation on expectation and emptiness," picturing a snowfall:

Then there is space ... Not emptiness, nor a lack of things, much less a memory of what was once there and desire for what could be. No, in that space, there's a rich possibility, an anything, an everything.[11]

The brain responds positively to open space—meadows of wild flowers, deserts that (at least from a distance) seem empty of everything but sand and light—and that can be metaphorical as well as literal. Think of the potential and excitement of a fresh notebook or a blank canvas. We've all experienced the rewards of a simple pause, a rest from stimulation. Despite what we might have been told as children, staring into "empty" space and daydreaming might in fact be time well spent.

Work with what you have

We can't all get to a farm or meadow, but even spending time in limited urban green space can have a positive effect. City-dwellers breathe in a lot of polluted air from cars and industry, filled with heavy metals such as arsenic and lead, and it creates inflammation, which harms the lungs and heart. Studies have shown that we can counter this and improve our lung tissue with a walk someplace green—a nearby park, your own backyard, the courtyard of your apartment complex, or a cul-de-sac ...

Being in a meadow, field, or any other open space brings many benefits, even if it's only *perceived* as an open space. The Construction Industry Research and Information Association (CIRIA), an advocate for green spaces in urban settings, supports what we learned from Ulrich in Chapter 1, that views of or access to green spaces can improve and hasten recovery from illness or surgery and lessen the need for medication. CIRIA goes on to say that research has shown that people who live near open spaces with some element of green "seem to be more effective in managing major life issues, coping with poverty, and performing better in cognitive tasks."[12]

Even walking through the city to a park or green area has been shown to calm our minds. In 2017, using EEGs, self-reported measures, and interviews, researchers at the universities of York and Edinburgh showed that, among the elderly, "Walking between busy urban environments and green spaces triggers changes in levels of excitement, engagement and frustration in the brain."[13]

Foraging

For those of us who do have access to the countryside, there is another kind of healing to be found where things grow wild. As Robin Wall Kimmerer wrote in *Braiding Sweetgrass: Indigenous Wisdom, Scientific Knowledge, and the Teachings of Plants* (2014), "Plants know how to make food and medicine from light and water, and then they give it away."[14] Foraging—not just in rural areas, but even in city parks—is becoming more popular, and is a way to be somewhere green and do some marketing for "free." Berries are a great example. According to the Irish botanist and medical biochemist (and personal hero of mine!) Diana Beresford-Kroeger, wild lingonberries, blackberries, elderberries, cloudberries, raspberries, and other small fruit carry "an extraordinary biochemical reward" called ellagic acid, which creates a filter that reduces the "mutagenicity" of toxins entering our cells.[15] This matters because mutagens are chemical or physical agents capable of causing genetic alterations or mutations and damaging DNA, leading to cancer and other illnesses.

Beyond berries, knowledgeable foragers can collect mushrooms, wild carrots, fern fiddleheads, and herbs such as wild mint and sage. They can even gather seaweed as we'll see in Chapter 8! My neighborhood still has remnants of the harvestable kitchen gardens that were there many years ago: an apple tree, a pear tree, a fig tree, plenty of mulberry trees, and some grapevines.

There are a couple of caveats, of course. First of all, know what you're putting into your mouth, especially when it comes to mushrooms, which can be highly poisonous. The best way to begin foraging is with someone who knows what they're doing. It may be a friend who has been living off their land for a long time, or someone who has dedicated themselves to studying the local flora. Look online for details of local foraging walks or groups. Second, consider the soil the plants are growing in, and make sure they haven't been exposed to toxic or bacteria-laden man- or animal-made substances.

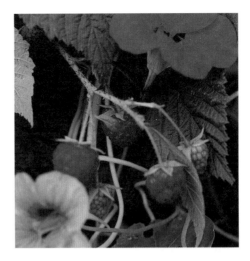

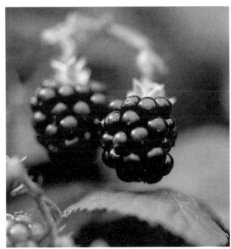

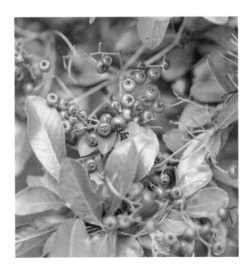

FOUR WAYS TO BRING
THE GARDEN INTO YOUR HOME

Sometimes you can get outside to nature, but a way to bring a little bit of nature to you is by growing some easy things. Those glimmers of green in pots on the windowsill boost our mood, and they can be nourishing, too. Here are some examples:

- **I always have a few scallions or spring onions sprouting,** and I use them all the time. They're really simple to cultivate. When you bring the onions home from the market, save the white root of two or three and put them in a glass with just enough water to cover the bulb. Leave them on a sunny windowsill and be sure to change the water every day or so, or it will become kind of funky. Then, when you need a little bit to flavor a salad or sauce, trim some off. You'll always have something fresh and green to eat, no matter the season. If you wish, plant the bulbs in your garden in spring, and they'll spread.

- **Once you start experimenting with things in glasses and jars on the windowsill,** you'll delight in what you can grow. I've always been a failure at rooting avocado pits, but when my son was small he loved it when we were able to start a pineapple plant by cutting the crown from the fruit, drying the stalk, and rooting it in sandy soil. It took a few months, but we actually harvested a tiny pineapple! This is a lovely way to have a little bit of Hawaii on your kitchen counter in January.

- **I discovered this one by accident when I was cutting back a mulberry tree in spring** before the berries started dropping onto the roof. The leafy stems were so lively and fresh that I rinsed them and put them in a vase. It had never occurred to me before to do this with flower-free cuttings, but now I do it all the time. The breath of green freshness without a corresponding plant to tend is always pleasing.

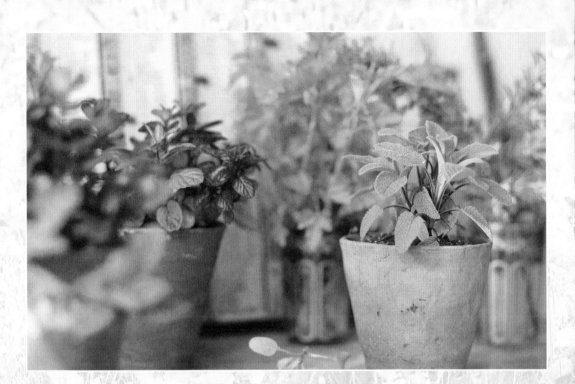

- **It was also in spring that I brought home my first batch of herbs from the farmers' market.** I had dill, sage, basil, and mint, and couldn't use them all at once. I'd read that herbs keep better in water than packed up and refrigerated, so I cleaned and trimmed them and put them in four matching glasses. I had sage that lasted almost a month this way. The effect and the fragrance were lovely, and no basil wilted or grew slimy in the back of the crisper. (Warning: my cats seem fascinated by dill and couldn't leave it alone, so I had to put it in an inaccessible spot!)

CHAPTER 6

THE SENSE OF NATURE

*I go to nature to be soothed and healed, and
to have my senses put in order.*

John Burroughs, 1837–1921

HEALING COLORS, PATTERNS, SCENTS, SOUND, AND SILENCE

Recent studies by the noted social scientist Peter Aspinall of Heriot-Watt University, Edinburgh, and his colleagues have demonstrated that walking through urban green space elevated brain electroencephalogram (EEG) readings, lowering frustration and heightening engagement, and had an especially healing impact on older adults.[1] One can't help but wonder whether this effect is caused by the absence of city stress or something else. Maybe it has more to do with what the subjects are seeing—the green—than with where they are?

In 1984, Dr. Roger Ulrich (see Chapter 1) published new research in *Science* that went beyond his initial breakthrough in the late 1970s that demonstrated the healing power of looking out of windows into green space.[2] In his new work, Ulrich reported even more remarkable results. Hospital patients who had plants in their rooms or even just looked at *photographs* of nature recovered much more quickly from surgery and required fewer painkillers. Perhaps this explains why we feel compelled to bring flowers to people who are sick. The blossoms brighten things up and immediately change the tone of the environment. They might be accompanied by a pleasing smell, but their uplifting effect seems to be primarily visual. As my neighbor Audra Tsanos, whose garden is a thing of wonder and delight in almost every season, puts it, "The eye seeks green." Nature produces a visual experience of infinite complexity and subtlety.

Seeing colors

When we look at an object, it reflects light, which is received by the cells in our retinas, producing messages that are interpreted by the brain as images, colors, intensity, and so on. In the back of the eye, rods process light and dark and cones process the varying wavelengths that are perceived as color. Our brains are directly affected by what we see; there is a short but critical path between our eyes and our brain, and different parts of the brain hold different information: faces, motion, distance, luminance. (We'll consider luminance in Chapter 8, and why spending too much time looking at screens can have negative effects.)

In her book *Healing Spaces*, Esther M. Sternberg asks: "Is there something about the structure of a scene that might be intrinsically jarring or relaxing—that could change your mood or affect healing?" She answers the question by explaining that there is a pathway from the visual cortex—the part of our brain that receives and processes sensory nerve impulses from the eyes—to the parahippocampal place area, which recognizes and recalls environmental scenes (such as landscapes) over other stimuli (such as faces). That's interesting, but this is amazing: "The nerve cells along this pathway express an increasing density of receptors of endorphins—the brain's own morphine-like molecules."[3]

Think of the possibilities: We might be able to heal ourselves simply by looking at images from nature! Sternberg goes on to explain how beautiful natural tableaux such as sunsets or misty forests have been shown to stimulate this opiating pathway. Remarkably, the more the nerve cells are stimulated by motion, color, and a variety of depths of perspective, the more active and opiating the release of endorphins becomes. Perhaps this evolved as a survival tool: the more that primitive people could see as they scanned the horizon, the more useful and potentially life-saving information they could gather. We have become what the neuroscientist Dr. Edward Vessel of the Max Planck Institute for Empirical Aesthetics calls "infovores," using visual information both to ascertain risk and to spark "cognitive pleasure."[4]

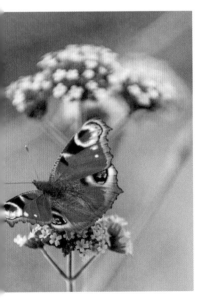 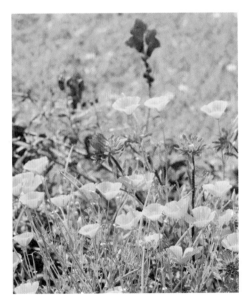 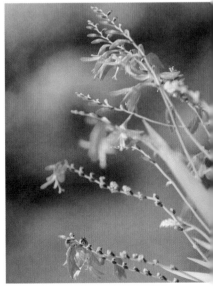

Not only green

Green is not the only color to which we have an instinctive reaction. The longer the wavelength of the colors we're looking at (reds and oranges, rather than blues), the better we think. Studies at Rockefeller University have shown that our alertness and cognitive abilities are enhanced when we are exposed to orange light, as opposed to blue, which has a shorter wavelength.[5] This might be why we may grow dreamier when looking at a blue sky, but are drawn to and thrilled by sunsets. Perhaps it's related to the colors of the sunrise, as well—the beacon of a new day.

Speaking of blue, the neurosurgeon Amir Vokshoor says that, because of its shorter wavelength, blue has a relaxing effect and tends to evoke a more positive emotional response, related to dopamine or the "feel-good" hormone. He wrote: "the arousal mechanism stimulated by blue's wavelengths correlates to the release of neurotransmitters thought to be associated with feelings of euphoria, joy, reward, and wellness."[6] It follows that, just as we need to eat

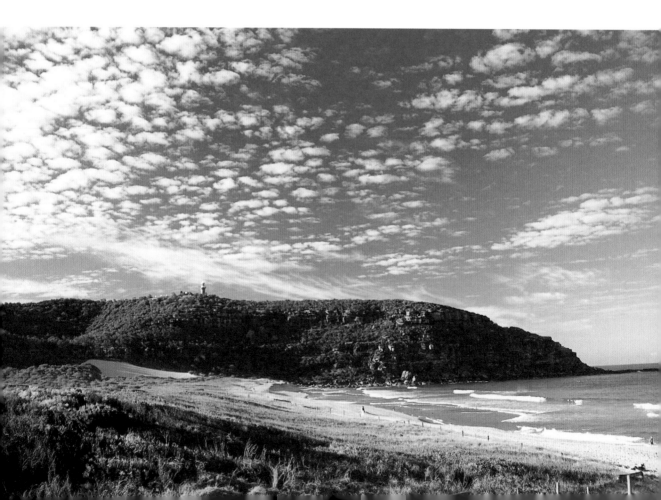

a variety of foods, we should make sure we have some exposure to natural light's full color spectrum every day (if possible) if we want to enhance our brain function and feel more alert and even happier.

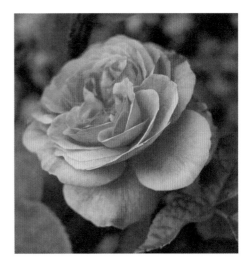

Stop and see the roses

A body of research undertaken by Japanese scientists in 2016 revealed a startling fact: that simply seeing fresh flowers (not even smelling or touching them) has benefits. Chorong Song and her colleagues assembled a group of 114 people of varying ages, genders, and occupations, and had each person look at a bouquet of thirty pink *odorless* roses for four minutes. By analyzing the participants' pulses, the scientists concluded that the visual stimulation of looking at the roses increased parasympathetic nervous activity, fostering a state of relaxation, while simultaneously decreasing sympathetic nervous activity and alleviating stress.[7] Think about that: Merely seeing flowers can calm us, and with that state of ease all sorts of healing—both physical and psychological—are more likely.

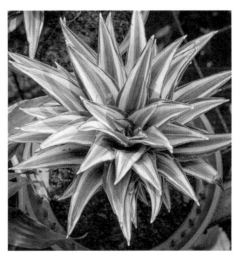

Further study produced similar results with striped *Dracaena* or corn plants, a common houseplant. And even more studies have shown that we experience a calming response from observing three-dimensional plants and flowers—even if they are artificial—in lieu of photographs.[8] In other words, the real thing is best, artificial the second best choice, but even photographs of fauna will produce some positive effects.

Fractals

Fractals are structures in which the same pattern recurs at a progressively smaller scale. Think about how the vein patterns of a leaf echo the appearance of the tree itself. The geometry of fractals is all around us—zoom in on a fern, a pine tree, a snowflake, a snail shell, a Queen Anne's lace flower, or a head of broccoli, and you'll find fractals. Dr. Qing Li (see Chapter 3) incorporates them into his forest bathing instructions, and writes that after gazing at fractals, first as light through a tree canopy and then as leaves, parts of leaves, and veins, we can appreciate the interconnected patterns of the natural world. With that appreciation can come sensations of wonder and delight, as well as of quietude and tranquility.[9]

Richard Taylor, professor of physics at the University of Oregon, is developing retinal implants to restore vision for people suffering from eye disease. In the process he looked at images of Jackson Pollock's action paintings. At first you might think this is a stretch—from Abstract Expressionist painting to inner eye implants—but it was through Pollock's art that Taylor first realized how nature's fractals might relate to human stress. Because of this, he made sure that the implants he developed simulated the retina's design to induce the same kind of stress reduction that would result when looking at nature's fractals through healthy eyes.

Taylor found that seeing fractals stimulates the pleasure centers in the brain, but it went further than that. When his team used EEGs to monitor electrical activity in the brain and electrical responses in the skin of their subjects, they found that looking at works of art—such as Pollock's paintings—produced a reduction in stress of 60%. *Sixty percent!* That's with no medication, no mantras, no stretches or yoga poses, just looking at a fractal-rich painting. They also discovered that the physiological change initiated by looking at the art accelerated recovery from surgery.[10] Mind-blowing!

The scents of nature

The green cure isn't just about vision, it's also about smells. A great many studies have explored how smell influences our thinking. In particular, essential oils and other forms of fragrance can have a positive effect on how we remember and pay attention, on our self-confidence and experience of pain, and on how

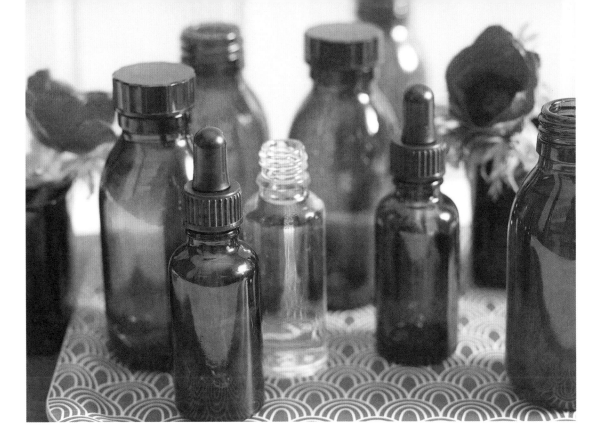

we make decisions.[11] This should sound pretty familiar to people who have tried aromatherapy, and there is a science to it. For example, it's been tested and shown that people who inhale the fragrance of rose oil feel calmer, more relaxed, and dreamier than those in a control group who don't. This has led to further research into the use of rose fragrance in treating or abating depression and anxiety.[12]

Of course, it's not just about roses. As we learned through forest bathing, the smell of pine woods and phytoncides—those volatile organic compounds that boost immune function—have a beneficial effect on our bodies and minds.

Sound

In her book *#What Is Sound Healing?* (2016), Lyz Cooper, founder of the British Academy of Sound Therapy, defines sound as audible energy. She goes on to say that "it is the result of particles of matter vibrating to make waves that are 'big' enough and of the right pitch to be audible to the human ear."[13] Then our brain makes sense of those vibrations and gives them meaning—a baby's cry, a jackhammer, a babbling brook. Too many sounds, or unpleasant ones, can have a deleterious effect.

According to a study undertaken in 2018 by the Brighton and Sussex Medical School (BSMS) in the south of England, hearing sounds from nature, such as the roar of the ocean, helps us to focus our attention and allows us to relax.[14] You're not making it up when you feel as though the burble of running water, sparrows chirping, or the rustling of prairie grass relaxes you.

BSMS collaborated with the audiovisual artist Mark Ware to study what happened when people listened to recordings of natural and artificial sounds. Using an MRI scanner, they gauged brain activity while monitoring infinitesimal changes in heart rate. They learned that natural sounds increased brain connectivity and directed attention outward, whereas artificial sounds focused attention inward, creating a state similar to anxiety, depression, or PTSD.[15] After all, I can't imagine that anyone wouldn't feel calmer listening to the rustling of trees or a stream than to traffic or construction sounds.

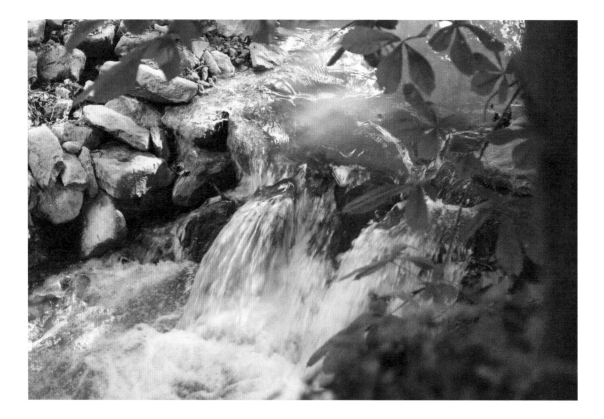

Even listening to natural sounds played on headphones increases parasympathetic activation, promoting and sustaining a sense of rest and counteracting stress. In a study published in the *International Journal of Environmental Research and Public Health* in 2010, university students exposed to natural sounds such as fountains and birdsong, rather than traffic noise, dealt better with a stressor (an arithmetic test).[16] There are long-term health benefits of diminished stress, so maybe it's time to dig out all those nature CDs or download a few tracks of whale calls or soothing rain rhythms—or maybe even record your own. Turn off your screens and try listening to sounds like this before going to sleep. (If you're in the city, try playing a recording at low volume.)

BIRDSONG

Birdsong has been found to be particularly restorative. Julian Treasure, author of *Sound Business* (2006), has said that birdsong evokes a state that he calls "body relaxed, mind alert." In 2013, he told the BBC: "People find birdsong relaxing and reassuring because over thousands of years they have learnt [that] when the birds sing they are safe, [and] it's when birds stop singing that people need to worry. Birdsong is also nature's alarm clock, with the dawn chorus signalling the start of the day, so it stimulates us cognitively." Treasure has put this to good use in a free smartphone app called Study, which claims to be a "productivity-boosting" soundscape to listen to while you work. He says it can help you to focus, improve cognition, and reduce tiredness. It's also intended to mask background noise—particularly conversation—that can disturb your concentration.[17]

Sound has such a potent effect on us that some people think we should be aware of it in the same way as we monitor what we eat, drink, or breathe. After all, it's effectively another substance that we're putting into our bodies.

SILENCE

Just as sounds can be healing, so is silence. Although it is hard to come by, most of us would agree that quiet is essential. Think about noise pollution, blaring screens, even the sometimes desirable background of white noise. All of it can lead to stress, sleeplessness, and more. We seek out earplugs and noise-canceling headphones for temporary respite, because it's easier to relax, think, and create without the stress and disruption of noise. Our world seems to be getting louder—with more traffic, cellphone pings and buzzes, televisions in waiting rooms, and music piped in everywhere—so seeking silence can be a challenge.

Traditional Japanese gardens include specific sense components, so that they address all means of perception, including sound. Running water is often incorporated, not just because it is perceived as cleansing, but also because its gentle sound contrasts with and enhances the silence.[18] How many times have you been able to solve a problem or clarify a situation after you've had a quiet moment to sort it out? That's where silence comes in, when the television is off, when you're all alone, or the moment at a crowded party or on a busy railroad station when suddenly everything falls still.

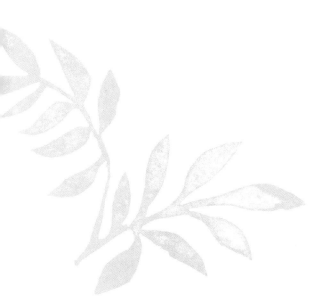

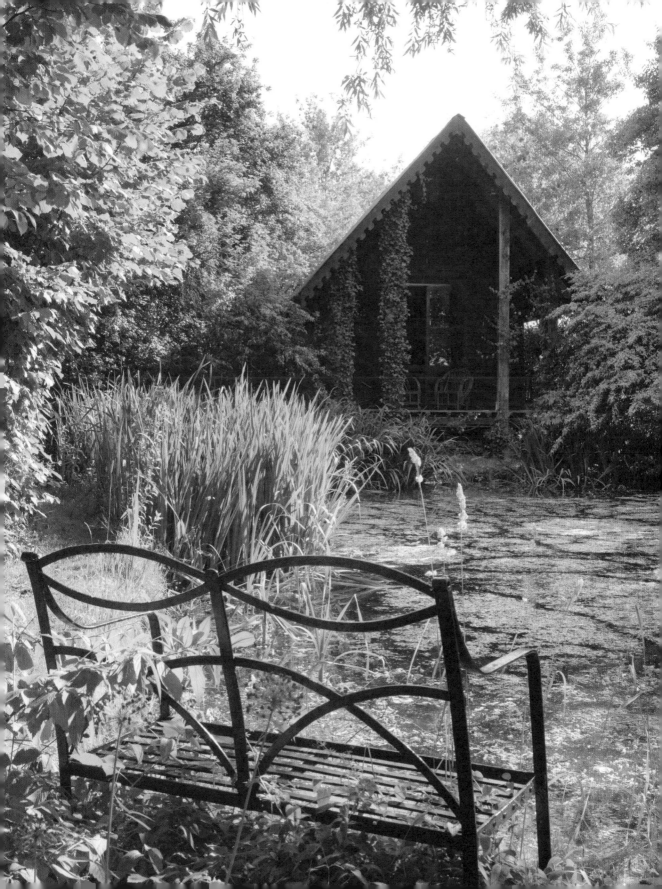

SENSE MEDITATION

In just the same way as we can focus on our breath and the sensations of our bodies, we can meditate on the sensations coming from the world around us. This can apply to any of our senses, and it is a form of mindfulness. There's a famous exercise popularized by Jon Kabat-Zinn and taught in Mindfulness Stress Reduction Programs using the contemplation and deliberate consumption of a single raisin to increase presence in mindfulness meditation.[19] For our purposes I've adapted it to a dandelion flower, but it could be anything from nature—a pine cone, a rose petal, a blade of grass. See if you experience some of the green cure effects of deeply experiencing a small bit of nature.

1. **Find a comfortable, quiet place to sit.** This might be your favorite park bench, near a window as the sun rises, or on a blanket in the garden. Wherever it is, make sure it's a spot that allows you to get as quiet and as connected as possible to some aspect of nature. If all else fails, play a recording of nature sounds.

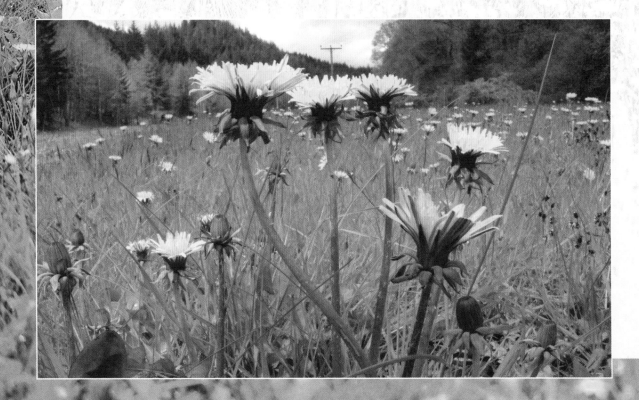

2. **Pause and assess how you feel.** Are you anxious? Tired? Restless? Bleary? Make a mental note of the sensation.

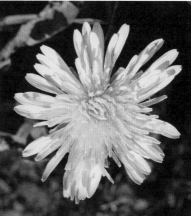

3. **Now, pick up the dandelion** or whatever you're using for your meditation and weigh it in the palm of your hand. Feel its heft or lightness. Is it soft? Sticky?

4. **Next, look at it.** Really focus on it with your complete attention. Imagine it's the first dandelion you've ever seen. Can you find any fractal patterns? What does the color yellow evoke for you?

5. **Turn the flower over between your fingers and connect to its texture and feel.** Try closing your eyes, so that all your information comes solely from touch.

6. **Try smelling the dandelion.** Is there a fragrance? Is it pleasant or unpleasant? Assuming you're not allergic, don't just sniff it, but hold it near your nose and breathe slowly and deeply. Repeat for a few breaths.

7. **Now, close your eyes and picture the dandelion.** What does it evoke for you? Look at that thought and let it go as you assess how you feel. Are you more relaxed? Focused? Do you feel more connected to your surroundings?

This kind of meditation practice gives a whole new meaning to the idea of taking time to stop and smell the flowers!

CHAPTER 7

FROM THUNDERSTORMS TO DESERT HEAT

*A change in the weather is sufficient
to recreate the world and ourselves.*

Marcel Proust, *In Search of Lost Time,*
The Guermantes Way (1920–21)

WEATHER CAN TRANSFORM US

We are more affected by the weather than simply needing to grab an overcoat when it's cold or search for an umbrella when it rains. In *The Weather Detective* (2018), Peter Wohlleben wrote that some of us have an internal barometer that responds to atmospheric pressure, which is why we experience arthritis and other sorts of pain when the pressure falls.[1] This is called meteor-sensitivity or weather sensitivity, and some experts believe that this discomfort occurs when air changes from warm and dry to cold and damp, lowering the sensitivity threshold of the nervous system.

The Japanese call it *tenki-tsu*, weather pains.[2] Jun Sato of Aichi Medical University, who researches the relationship between pain and weather and what causes it, has found that when the weather is inclement and the atmospheric pressure falls, people experience more stress. That's because our bodies respond to the pressure by activating the autonomic nervous system, which causes blood pressure to rise and pulse to increase, leading to chronic pain (especially joint pain) as well as migraines and emotional troubles such as anxiety.

The weather even affects our posts on social media! Scientists who examined data from social media posts to see how weather related to emotion found that temperature, precipitation, humidity, and cloud cover were associated with:

- Self-expression—both positive and negative;
- An increase of positive comments when the temperature was up to 70°F (20°C), and a decline as it rose above 86°F (30°C);
- Negative comments when it was raining, especially on days when the humidity was 80% or higher, as well as on very cloudy days.[3]

The short version? People are happier and friendlier when the weather is good.

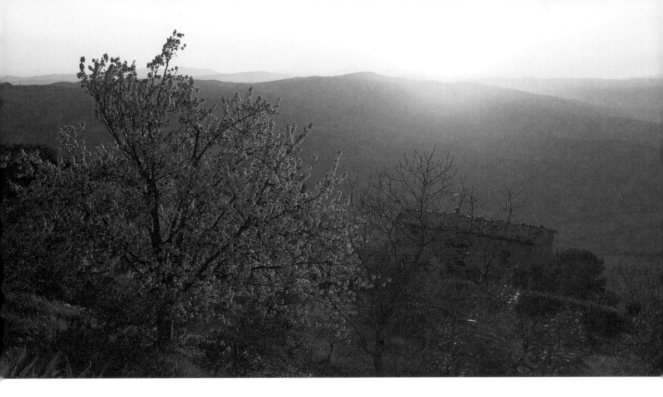

Sunshine

As we learned in Chapter 1, vitamin D is the sunshine vitamin. We need it to build healthy bones and teeth, and also to:

- Support the health of the immune system, brain, and nervous system;
- Regulate insulin levels and aid our management of diabetes;
- Support lung function and cardiovascular health;
- Slow the rate of cancer progression.[4]

The best way to get vitamin D is through exposure to unfiltered sunlight, and there are other benefits to spending time in the sun as well. Regular exposure to sunlight under a physician's guidance:

- Helps to abate atherosclerosis, the buildup of deposits that can clog arteries and lead to coronary heart disease;[5]
- May be an effective means of slowing the development of obesity;[6]
- May prevent or diminish inflammatory diseases of the liver;[7]
- Can facilitate healing, from wounds to tuberculosis;[8]
- Can be part of a treatment for skin ailments including psoriasis, acne, and rosacea;[9]
- Can affect insomnia and how well we sleep (see Chapter 9).

Aim for ten to fifteen minutes at midday (between 10 a.m. and 3 p.m. depending on time zone), three days per week. Be sure not to overdo it, though: You can have too much of a good thing, and overexposure to sunlight can lead to maladies ranging from heat exhaustion to skin cancer.

SOLAR STORMS

Solar or geomagnetic storms occur when the sun releases a huge burst of energy into the cosmos in the form of electrons, ions, and atoms, along with the usual electromagnetic waves. The most highly charged storms can affect our wellbeing here on Earth. Research published in the *Proceedings of the Royal Society* found that such storms may disorientate our hormonal systems and those of other mammals, affecting behavior and health.[10] This disorientation may lead to anxiety, fatigue, difficulty in focusing, flu-like symptoms, and perhaps even increased psychic awareness.

It's hard to predict solar storms, unless you have a friend at NASA, but you can visit the websites of NASA or the American National Oceanic and Atmospheric Administration for information. If you find yourself suffering from some of the symptoms and think a storm may be the cause, here are a few things you can do:

- Drink plenty of filtered water (not tap water);
- Take saltwater baths;
- Meditate and remain aware of recurring thoughts and feelings;
- Avoid caffeine and alcohol;
- Spend time in nature (we knew that one already!);
- Remind yourself that everything in the universe is made up of energy, and that conscious thought and intention can instantly alter how we think and feel;
- Temporarily disconnect from technology if possible, and from anything or anyone toxic or draining.[11]

Spring fever?

It's a real thing! Although not a defined medical condition, it's certainly more than a subject for poets or a catalyst for students to fidget at their desks. According to Dr. Michael Terman, professor of clinical psychology in psychiatry at Columbia University, when the snow melts and the days grow longer and warmer, spring fever starts with mood swings and surges into a burst of energy that contrasts with our slower, steadier state of mind during the winter.[12] It's likely because the days are longer and we get more light, and it's why we have a better outlook and more vitality, and may even be motivated to do some spring cleaning!

Spring fever also brings to mind the opening moments of the movie *Bambi*, with bunnies and deer frolicking and falling in love. Animals tend to mate in the spring so that they'll have a rich food source for their offspring throughout summer and autumn. And it might not be just woodland creatures, either: Professor Nicolas Guéguen of the University of South Brittany, France, discovered that the women he studied tended to be a little more open to romance on sunny days. More than a fifth, or 22.4%, gave out their phone numbers on fine days, as opposed to 13.9% when the weather was cloudy.[13]

The coming of spring has an impact on learning, too. Children tend to be more receptive to ideas and more energetic—perhaps because sunshine increases levels of dopamine—the neurotransmitter that regulates

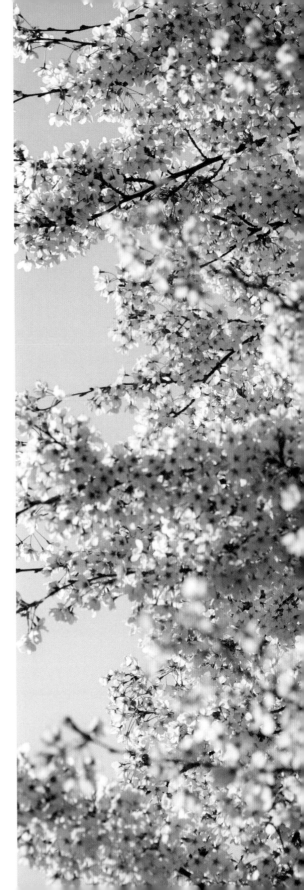

the brain's pleasure and reward centers. Although I think most students' first reaction is to want to be sprung from the classroom with the coming of good weather, teachers can direct that boost in mood and enthusiasm for learning and retaining new information.[14]

Singing in the rain

Sunny days have their benefits, but so do rainy ones. Rain is not just good for vegetable crops or the flower garden, it is good for our minds as well. As the health writer Denise Mann puts it, "negative ions create positive vibes."[15] Negative ions are oxygen ions with an extra electron attached, and can result from changes in weather conditions, so when it rains they're produced through water molecules, which is why they are plentiful in rainstorms, at the beach, and near waterfalls. This is one of the reasons that taking a shower or bath refreshes us and reduces fatigue. Standing outside or even just opening the window during a downpour provides us with the benefit of negative ions and increases the flow of oxygen to the brain, producing biochemical reactions that raise serotonin, improving our mood and making us more alert. Other studies report that negative ions can facilitate the treatment of PTSD, addiction, and depression.[16] They may also filter out dust, easing allergies and even asthma.

THE PERFUME OF RAIN

Why is it that the smell of rain makes us feel so good? Scientists have been studying this since the 1960s, when two Australian researchers, Isabel "Joy" Bear and Richard Grenfell Thomas, coined the term "petrichor," meaning "a distinctive scent, usually described as earthy, pleasant, or sweet, produced by rainfall on very dry ground."[17] As reported in the *Smithsonian Magazine*, theirs and later research determined that a primary cause of this fragrance is the combination of oils discharged by some plants during dry weather. Compounds of these oils accumulate on dry rocks and soil, and when good, heavy rain comes, they mix and discharge into the air. Bear and Grenfell hypothesized that this had to do with when seeds germinated, and that plants produced them almost as a kind of birth control to prevent germination during drought, when there wouldn't be enough water to nourish the seedlings.[18]

All this is fascinating, but still, why do we like the smell so much? The anthropologist Diana Young, who studies the culture of Western Australia's Pitjantjatjara people, has noted that they connect the petrichor with the color green, perhaps indicating a primal connection between rainy season and the promise of vegetation and game and the sustenance they bring. She has named this phenomenon "cultural synesthesia," or "the blending of different sensory experiences on a society-wide scale due to evolutionary history."[19] This linking of smell to memory brings us back to how deeply and intrinsically we're connected to green.

Not so positive

Just as negative ions make us feel better, positive ones can make us feel worse. Think how weary you become in an airless, stuffy classroom or in a car with the windows closed. But not all fresh air has a positive effect. When wind flows through an arid area, the dust it picks up leeches the positive ions, creating what are sometimes called "witches' winds," "evil winds," or "devil winds," such as the Santa Ana in California, the *foehn* in the European Alps, the *hamsin* or *khamsin* in Israel, and the chinook in the Rockies. All have been known to affect people deeply, making them irritable, nasty, and mean-tempered, and this is probably because of the positive ions, according to the psychiatrist and scientist Norman E. Rosenthal.[20] (Rosenthal was the first to name Seasonal Affective Disorder, which we'll look at in the next chapter.)

These "evil" winds, which also include the *sirocco* of Italy, the *ghibli* of Libya, and the *zonda* of the Argentine Andes, don't just provoke unpleasant feelings, they've also been associated with increased anxiety, crime, and suicide. There is a lot of anecdotal evidence to support this (talk to anyone in Los Angeles in the fall and you'll get an earful about what it's like to breathe air desiccated by the Santa Ana), but little scientific work has been done in this area, except for an often-quoted study by Willis H. Miller in 1968, correlating crime and evil winds.[21] It is a subject that would bear more research.

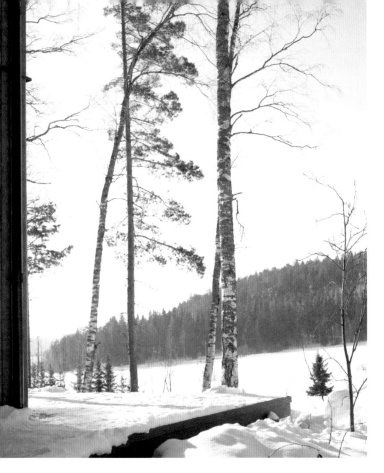

Hibernation

Winter has a bad reputation, but despite the boots and the heating bills, it does have positive effects. The longer nights and the fact that our mobility is limited by ice and snow allow us to rest more and sleep for longer. Being stuck indoors and watching snow fall has been described by some as a meditative or contemplative experience. Even without the cardio workout of shoveling, snow brings health benefits that help us to weather the dark days. Exposing the body to cold temperatures (cryotherapy) can raise our levels of norepinephrine, a chemical in the nervous system that may play a role in lessening pain.[22]

In Russian and Scandinavian countries, it is quite common to see babies napping outdoors in their strollers, even when the weather is very cold. Research by Marjo Tourula of the University of Finland found that leaving infants (carefully bundled in warm clothing) outside to sleep in really cold weather not only promotes better sleep, but also increases the length of the nap. The parents she interviewed believed that napping in the fresh air promoted health in their infants, helping them to grow hearty and develop resistance to disease, especially colds.[23] Parents keep an eye on their babies and do not let them get over-chilled, and in Sweden they subscribe to the saying, "There is no bad weather, just bad clothing."

But is it a dry heat?

Hot weather isn't all bad, either. Spending time in the desert or other hot, dry places can be a way to get a rich dose of sunshine and can be of benefit to both muscles and lungs. Desert air tends to be some of the least contaminated by air pollution, because there's less human activity, and it is the best for allergy sufferers, because there's very little pollen in such a barren environment.

If you're an athlete, training in the desert can significantly up your game. According to Santiago Lorenzo, a professor of physiology at Lake Erie College of Osteopathic Medicine and a former decathlete, besides increasing perspiration, exercising in heat can increase the volume of blood plasma (leading to improved cardiovascular fitness), lower the core temperature, and improve other indicators, leading to a better workout than in cool temperatures. Training in hot weather might even be a better way to stimulate physiological adaption than the traditional practice of improving training efficiency by doing it at high altitude.[24] High-temperature workouts may not be a regimen for the average person, but with acclimation, proper hydration, and supervision the benefits can be huge. If you're preparing for a marathon or tennis match, you might want to look into it.

Even those of us who live far from the desert can benefit from dry heat by going to a sauna. Most gyms and health clubs have them, and mobile saunas have become popular in big cities, allowing people to take in some heat close to home. The sweat is worth it: A Finnish study found that regular sauna bathing is associated with a reduced risk of sudden cardiac arrest, coronary heart disease, and fatal cardiovascular disease, and brings more general health benefits, too.[25] The Finns know a thing or two about saunas, after all. It's a huge part of their culture, and there are approximately 2 million saunas among a population of almost 5.5 million, which means one for every two or three people![26]

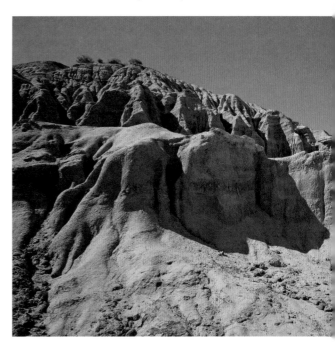

SUN SALUTATIONS

Pretty much anyone who has taken a yoga class has encountered sun salutations. They are best done in the morning, and can be calibrated for difficulty according to your ability. They are thought to awaken the energy of our inner sun or core as it stretches and flexes our muscles, stimulating our joints and organs and increasing blood flow.

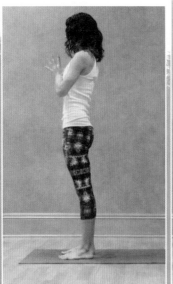

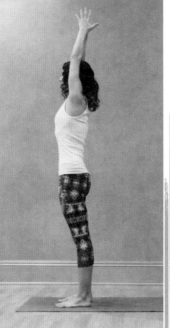

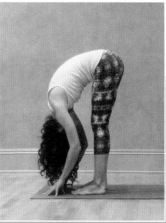

1 Stand with your feet parallel, feeling connected to the ground. Bring your palms together and release your shoulders.

2 Take a deep breath and raise your arms overhead, bringing your palms together.

3 Release your breath and your arms as you bend forward. Keep your legs as straight as you can, but don't lock your knees. Feel the weight of your head as it hangs down.

But have you ever tried doing sun salutations outdoors? In the heat on a beach? On a misty spring morning? On an early winter's day before the first snowfall? Try it. (It is said that doing 108 rounds of sun salutations is especially auspicious. Good luck!) Here is a simplified version of the sun salutations that are taught in most yoga classes:

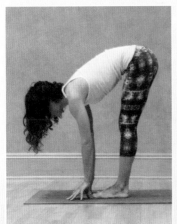

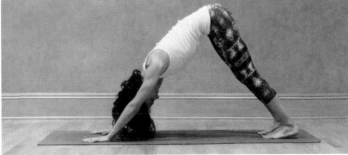

5 Step your right foot back, followed by your left foot, putting your feet together into a downward dog. Exhale, and feel yourself connected to the earth.

4 Inhale and send your fingertips down to the ground, straighten your elbows, and lift your torso away from your thighs. Stretch your entire spine.

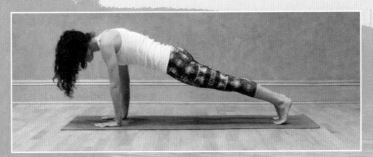

6 Move into plank pose. Inhale and bring your torso forward until your shoulders are above your wrists, arms perpendicular to the floor.

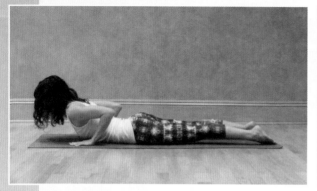

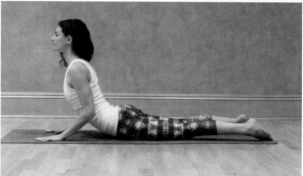

7 Breathe out as you lower your knees and then torso to the floor, bending your elbows as you do so. Look down at the floor or slightly ahead.

8 Inhale, straighten your arms slightly, and open your chest forward. With toes tucked under your feet, press your front thighs upward. Open your solar plexus— expand and stretch your chest sideways—as you look forward or up at the sky.

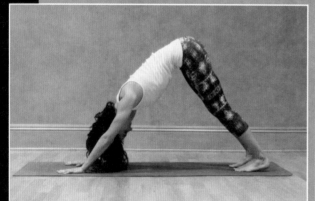

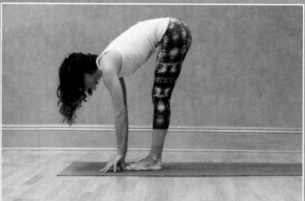

9 Release the breath as you move back into downward dog.

10 Inhale and send your fingertips down to the ground, straighten your elbows, and lift your torso away from your thighs. Stretch your entire spine.

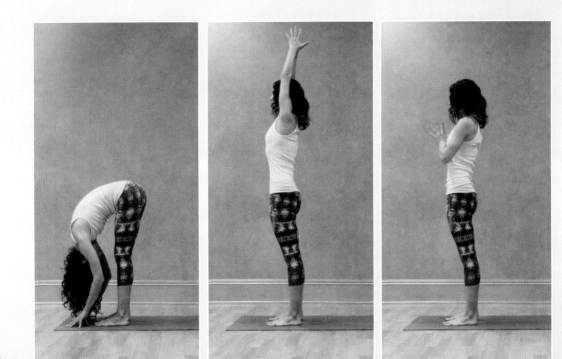

11 Exhale back into a forward fold.

12 Breathe in deeply and raise your arms overhead, bringing your palms together.

13 Exhale as you lower your arms and bring your palms together. This is one cycle.

When you have completed your sun salutations, rest on the ground if possible, or in a comfortable seated position. As you do, note your connection to the atmosphere, to the weather. What remains the same? What has changed?

CHAPTER 8

WATER TREATMENT

Water purifies and regenerates because it nullifies the past, and restores—even if only for a moment—the integrity of the dawn of things.[1]

Mircea Eliade, *Patterns in Comparative Religion* (1958)

PUDDLES TO OCEANS, SKIN TO BRAIN CHEMISTRY

People are drawn to the sea for respite and restoration, but we're also dependent on water. Human beings can live for about three weeks without food (if we really must), but usually less than a week without water.[2] Water performs most of our crucial physiological functions, including regulating our body temperature, building cells, metabolizing and digesting food, lubricating joints, carrying nutrients and oxygen to our cells, and flushing out toxins.[3] We are about 60% water, and it makes up about 31% of our bones and about 73% of our heart and brains.[4] The earliest life forms began in water, and, in some ways, because it's such a major part of our physiology, we never left it.

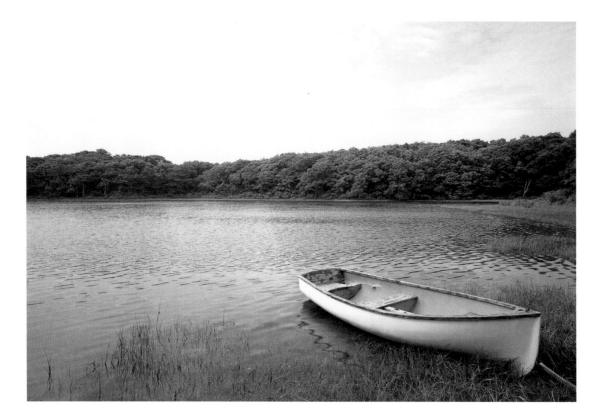

Drinking water

Get the best water you can, and drink it! Even increasing your water consumption by 1% (*one percent!*) can lower your daily caloric intake as well as your consumption of fat, sugar, salt, and cholesterol.[5] Those of us who have access to potable water have a remarkable healing elixir at our disposal, and we mustn't take it for granted. When it comes to water, obviously the cleaner and purer the better, and if you're doubtful about your water, boiling it for three minutes should kill most pathogens.[6] I avoid water that comes in plastic bottles for a few reasons:

- According to many reports, unless the source is specified, much bottled water is just packaged tap water.

- I'm concerned about chemicals in the plastic that may leach into the water, particularly BPA (bisphenol A), an industrial chemical used to make many kinds of plastic. It has been linked to heart disease, asthma, and diabetes, among other ailments, and is especially risky for children. When bottled water is the only option seek out BPA-free plastics, metal, or glass.

- Bottled water has often been found to have a higher level of bacteria than tap water, and it seems to me those transparent plastic bottles work as efficient bacteria incubators when left out in the sun.[7]

- Those plastic bottles are wasteful and often irresponsible because they seldom recycle effectively, yet they must go somewhere—landfills or, worse, our oceans. Ultimately, the green cure relies on our planet being healthy.

Seeing the sea

Our need for water is about more than just staying hydrated. We're endlessly fascinated by and connected to it. For example, some 270 million visits are made to English coastlines each year, which is remarkable for a country with a population of 66 million.[8] As Wallace J. Nichols, founder of Ocean Revolution, wrote in his brilliant *Blue Mind: The Surprising Science that Shows How Being Near, In, On, or Under Water Can Make You Happier, Healthier, More Connected, and Better at What You Do* (2014), "water is changing all the time, but it's also fundamentally familiar. It seems to entertain our brains nicely with novelty plus a soothing regular background."[9]

Numerous scientific studies support the idea that just being near a body of water, like being near a green space, is good for body and mind. For example, analysis in 2012 by the University of Exeter found that the closer people lived to the coast, the healthier they tended to be. The researchers also learned that—as with green spaces—the positive impact was especially notable among less affluent socio-economic groups who have fewer opportunities to live near the sea or take holidays there, leading them to find a correlation between life near the shore, lowered stress, and increased exercise.[10]

Dr. Ulrich, whom we've come to know quite well by now, applied his research to views of greenery (see Chapter 1), but others have followed his lead and considered how seeing water scenes or "blue" environments can affect our health. Researchers at the universities of Exeter and Plymouth studied the physical and psychological effects of urban (gray), park and woodland (green), and river and coastline (blue) views on post-menopausal women as they rode stationary bikes for fifteen minutes.[11] The affective results—mood and feelings—for the green scenes were similar to those found by our friend Ulrich, and generally low for the urban environments (no surprise there), but the cyclists who were looking at blue scenes reported that the time seemed to go faster and they were more willing to keep exercising.[12]

Fortunately for the 60% of us who don't live near a coastline, even periodic visits can help us to flourish.[13] Researchers from Kobe University in Japan affirm that we humans thrive in natural environments and that visits to them can reduce stress and provide a sense of restoration, healing the body as we heal the mind. They also found that merely living near the beach isn't as helpful as stopping to take the time to appreciate the ocean view. Interestingly, there is a bigger impact on women than on men. Their experience of gazing at the sea induced feelings of grandeur, awe, peace of mind, and enchantment.

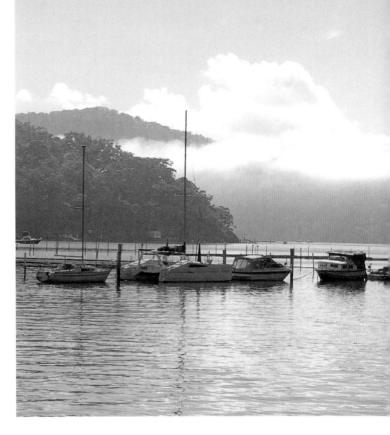

If you don't have the opportunity to take a beach holiday, don't worry: Scientists have linked this understanding to aquariums as well as to ocean views.[14] Research was conducted at the National Marine Aquarium in Plymouth, southern England, to find out if looking at biota (plant and animal life) in water affected physical and psychological wellbeing. The heart rate and mood of visitors to the aquarium were monitored as they looked at tanks containing only seawater, at partially stocked tanks, and at fully stocked tanks of fish and marine vegetation. One of the researchers, Dr. Mathew P. White, pointed out: "The first thing to notice is that people relaxed, even watching an empty tank, and the benefits increased as we introduced more fish."[15] This response was especially positive when it came to lowering stress. So, even if you live far from the sea, consider making regular visits to your local aquarium or setting up an aquatic tank of your own. If you have a challenging time keeping fish alive (as my son and I did when we tried it), think about growing aquatic plants instead—varieties of water fern are said to be quite easy—and skipping the fish altogether.

Seaweed

Fun fact: seaweed is a kind of algae, not a plant. It is high in protein, and contains vitamin B12, iodine, potassium, phosphorus, magnesium, sodium, and calcium.[16] Each of these is beneficial. Among other things, B12 encourages cell growth, iodine influences nerve and muscle function, potassium and sodium balance fluids in the body, phosphorus and calcium build bones and teeth, and magnesium regulates blood pressure. You can use seaweed for all sorts of things: It's a nutritious mulch for plants, great for thickening soups and seasoning stocks and salads, and can be a natural source of MSG, that savory *umami* taste. I like to smash it into tiny flakes, not quite a powder, and use it in rice instead of salt.

Consider foraging for your own! Ocean seaweed is generally safe to consume—whereas most freshwater algae are toxic—but there are a few exceptions, such as lyngbya, featherweed, and acid kelp. There are more than 35,000 types of seaweed, so do some research and be absolutely certain what you're putting in your mouth or on your skin. (If you're in doubt, opt for another green cure!)

Three abundant, accessible, and easy options found in the Atlantic Ocean are laver, giant kelp, and sea lettuce.[17] I tried harvesting laver—which is similar to nori that is used in sushi and Japanese snacks—because it seemed the least

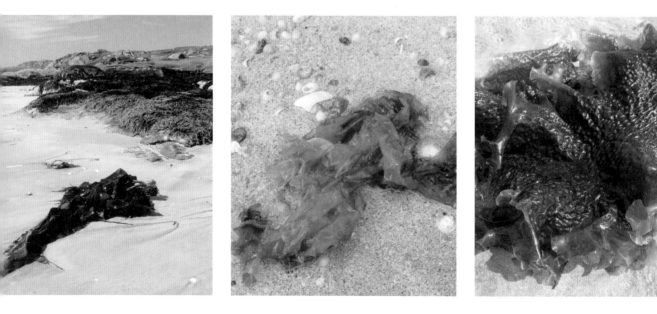

intimidating, and its dark green color made it easy to spot. It's best to harvest seaweed in cooler weather, because by summer it's at the end of its growing season and the heat can cause it to rot. Then:

- Make sure you're gathering from water that is unpolluted.
- Harvest living plants, not the seaweed that has washed ashore and is on the beach.
- Cut about 3–5 in. (7.5–12.5 cm) from the base.
- Wash thoroughly and as soon as possible (to free up any little sea creatures).
- Hang on a clothesline or drying rack in the sun for a few hours. It solidifies quickly!
- When it's thoroughly dry, store it in a humidity-proof container.

You can use nori as a face mask, as well as eating it, since it's said to be detoxifying. I tried this with the packaged dried sheets you can get at most health food or Asian specialty stores, but you could use foraged if you're feeling ambitious. Then:

- Moisten the seaweed in warm water.
- Apply to your face, close your eyes, and imagine you're on a beach holiday.
- Leave on for about 15 minutes.
- Wash off. If your skin tends toward dryness, apply a little more moisturizer than normal.

If you're feeling ambitious, add other components to your mask—like kelp, chlorella, aloe, or coconut oil—but be sure to experiment on a small patch of skin on your arm before putting it on your face.

Getting your feet wet

If you're at the beach—whether you're harvesting seaweed or not—think about taking off your shoes and socks and getting your feet wet. We all know that standing at the edge of the sea and feeling the cool waves lap at our feet is soothing, and so is the cooling sensation of walking through a cold mountain stream or a clear lake. Most of us have experienced the relief that comes from soaking our feet after a long day of standing or exercising.

Footbaths can soothe muscles and joints, but it turns out they may also ease our minds. Three times a week for four weeks, Japanese researchers gave footbaths and leg massages to psychiatric patients with schizophrenia,

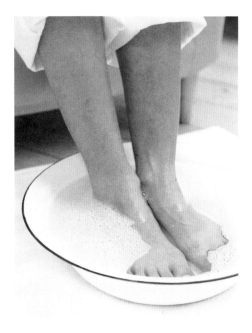

and measured the effects. The patients became more physically relaxed, which probably won't be a shock to most people. But what's fascinating is that the treatment was also successful in ameliorating their psychiatric symptoms.[18]

In a study of young women who were students at a nursing college in Nagano, Japan, a test was done to see what the effect of adding essential oil of lavender to footbath water had on the autonomic nervous system, the network responsible for our unconscious bodily functions, such as heartbeat, digestion, and breathing.[19] The women soaked their feet for ten minutes both with and without the lavender oil. The parasympathetic—calmer, "rest and digest"—nerve activity increased, regardless of whether the water had oil in it or not, even without the benefit of leg massage.

Take the plunge

If you're near a body of water, try taking a dip or a glide. It's common knowledge that swimming is great exercise, and so are boating or paddleboarding. When we're on a board or in a kayak, not only are we moving our muscles and strengthening our lungs, we're also applying mental focus to stay upright—improving balance and concentration—and we're directly connected to the psychological healing of being with water.

If you don't have a boat or a wetsuit, or the time to gather the equipment, try walking in water: It's better exercise than walking on land, because we're working against the water's resistance. This form of exercise is especially recommended for people with arthritis or limited abilities, for whom swimming laps is not a possibility. Plus, your feet get a nice massage as a bonus!

Bathing

Since time began, humans have been taking baths. The Romans built elaborate *thermae*, the ancient equivalent of the modern gym, with exercise rooms, massages, and heated water for cleaning and soaking. Many of these structures—the Baths of Caracalla in Rome, the eponymous Bath in England, and Varna in Bulgaria—still exist. Other cultures have followed suit, and the Japanese, Turks, and Swedes historically all had, and still have, elaborate bathing systems.

To bathe in nature, consider visiting a hot spring if you can. From Yellowstone National Park in the United States to the healing waters of Safaga, Egypt, Salar de Uyuni, Bolivia, or Antsirabe, Madagascar, immersion in warm, mineral-laden water has been shown to heal or ease muscle and joint pain, including arthritis, and to alleviate eczema and other skin conditions, and digestive disorders, especially when it's rich in sulfur.

Sometimes baths are used to heal the spirit, and pilgrims trek to water sources across the globe. Devotees of the Virgin Mary journey to partake of spring water in Lourdes, France, which they believe will heal their ills; millions of Muslims stop at the Well of Zamzam in Saudi Arabia while performing the hajj to Mecca; and Hindus seek out the Ganges River in India for spiritual purification. The ability of some these waters to heal us physically may come from their beneficial mineral content or soothing temperature, but no matter the pilgrim's destination or aspiration, there's something to be said for shared belief in a cure and a community directed toward a common effort.

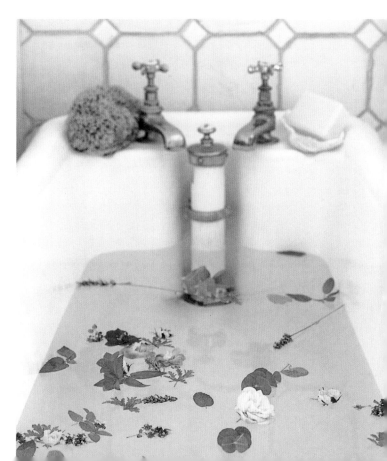

Even if you can't travel, there are plenty of good things about taking a bath in the comfort of your own home. Immersing yourself in water can be relaxing—think a warm soak after a long day, or a cooling dip in a lake on a summer's afternoon. It's commonly used after working out to prevent muscle stiffness, but it may also be an effective method of pain relief.[20] Tom B. Mole of the University of Cambridge and his colleagues have found that a quick swim in icy water may ease persistent pain after surgery almost as well as analgesics or physiotherapy. Although more research is needed, it's possible that the shock of diving into cold water stimulates the sympathetic ("fight or flight") nervous system, causing the body to respond to the sensation of cold instead of to that of pain, thus providing relief. Perhaps by overshadowing the pain with this frigid blast, the cycle is broken. This could be especially helpful for nerve pain, which is notoriously difficult to treat.

It even turns out that hot baths may be a way to receive some of the positive benefits of exercise. Scientists at Loughborough University compared the impact of an hour-long soak in a hot bath (104°F/40°C) on metabolic fitness and calories burned with that of an hour of cycling.[21] It turns out that although cycling burns more calories than bathing, the hot baths still resulted in the equivalent caloric output of a half-hour walk—about 140 calories! Hot baths also lowered blood sugar after eating and, more importantly, seemed to lower chronic inflammation, the body's response to infection, wounds, and diabetes.

Or you can try both. Alternating hot and cold baths is the foundation of a technique called contrast bathing, which is especially popular in Iceland and Scandinavia. The effect of immersing oneself in hot water and then cold, like having a cold dip after a sauna, is similar in principle to alternating hot and cold packs after an injury. The hot water increases blood flow throughout the body, while the cold constricts blood vessels, increasing local blood circulation in individual muscles.[22] Alternating hot and cold may also increase lymphatic flow and even improve the function of the immune system.[23]

Some of this positive effect isn't from the temperature at all, but from the gentle pressure of being under water, so choose whichever method works best for you.[24]

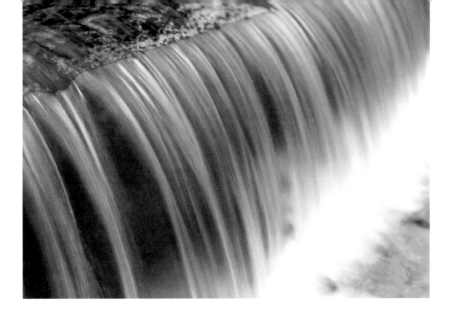

Chasing waterfalls

Remember negative ions, the oxygen molecules we read about in Chapter 7 that make us feel so good after rain? According to researchers from Paracelsus Medical University in Salzburg, Austria, a wonderful way to get a generous dose of those positive vibes is by visiting a waterfall, especially one at high altitude.[25] The falling water amps up the ionization, creating an aerosol effect that has positive psychological effects, lowering stress, and boosts the immune system. So, if you're fortunate enough to live near Iguaçu, Vitoria, Niagara, or Angel Falls, or even if you come across a mountain stream with a small descent while you are out forest bathing, make sure to spend some time nearby and experience the benefits!

Even thinking about that wonderful sound of rushing water is relaxing. I've heard people hypothesize that it's because it replicates the sound we hear in the womb. It may also be because our brains interpret sounds as threats (think thunder or alarm clocks) or comforts (think summer rain or waves lapping at the shore), according to Orfeu Buxton, an associate professor of biobehavioral health at Pennsylvania State University. Repeated soothing sounds create a sense of ease, he explains: "It's like they're saying: 'Don't worry, don't worry, don't worry.'"[26]

WATER MEDITATION

You don't need to live near the ocean or even know how to swim to find healing through water. Consider adding a water meditation to your selfcare practice.

My Zen teacher and friend Bonnie Myotai Treace of Hermitage Heart in Asheville, North Carolina, teaches a simple and beautiful water-bowl meditation. She describes it as "a way of shaping mind and heart, recognizing our intimacy with life."

- Fill a small bowl with water.
- Put it in a place that is meaningful to you—an altar if you have one, or on the sill of a window with a favorite view, or even on your desk.
- Top up the bowl whenever it gets low, or every day if you're not in a situation where water is scarce. Some people use snow in winter.
- Every time you fill the bowl, think about these words: *I offer this fresh water in recognition that my body and the body of all things are water. We are one thing even as we are different expressions. I vow to live this day in this wisdom, with kindness and generosity.*

If you'd like to experiment with something more elaborate, try a water-bowl offering based on a traditional Tibetan technique, taught by a Buddhist teacher trained in a Tibetan lineage and whom I work with and admire, Dr. Miles Neale.

- Gather seven small bowls or containers.
- Arrange them on an altar or in a place that has meaning for you, in a line, separated one from the other by the length of a grain of rice.
- Hold one of the bowls, fill it with water, and present it as an offering.
- Pour water from the first bowl into the second, from the second into the third, and so on. As you do, imagine you're transforming the liquid step-by-step into sacred materials:

1. Water to refresh
2. Water to bathe
3. Flowers to delight
4. Incense to perfume
5. Light to illuminate
6. Scented oil to ease
7. Food to nourish.

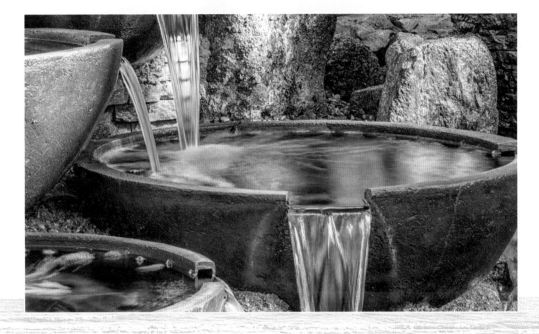

If you wish, you can incorporate sounds—music, affirmation, prayers, or mantra—or a candle to symbolize bringing light into the world.

Neale explains that the idea behind this practice "is based on the science of karmic causality—cause and effect—not dogma or rote. The power of creative imagination to influence our neurobiology is well documented, and so an ordinary act of offering water can be transformed into an extraordinary act of offering sacred substances. The brain registers the potency whether the action is real or imagined. The ritual then becomes a sacred skill training of openheartedness that optimally changes your mind and affects future perception."

Or, simply sit by your favorite body of water or even look at a glass of tap water, and meditate on these words, often attributed to the Lebanese-American poet Kahlil Gibran: "In one drop of water are found all the secrets of the oceans."

CHAPTER 9

CIRCADIAN RHYTHMS

*It is the unqualified result of all my experience
with the sick, that second only to their need
of fresh air is their need of light.*

Florence Nightingale, *Notes on Nursing* (1859)

MOONLIGHT, SUNSHINE, AND MINDFUL SLEEP

We spend a third of our lives sleeping or trying to fall asleep. Matthew Walker, director of the Center for Human Sleep Science at the University of California, Berkeley, studies brain activity to find out why we sleep, and what happens while we're sleeping and dreaming. He defines a lack of sleep as getting six hours or less per night, and believes that most of us spend our days in an "underslept" state. The consequences of this can be dire, he says, as "short sleep predicts a shorter life."[1] He goes on to explain that pretty much every disease people in developed nations suffer from is somehow linked to a substantial sleep deficit.

Walker isn't exaggerating. Sleep deprivation can lead to all kinds of symptoms and afflictions, such as:

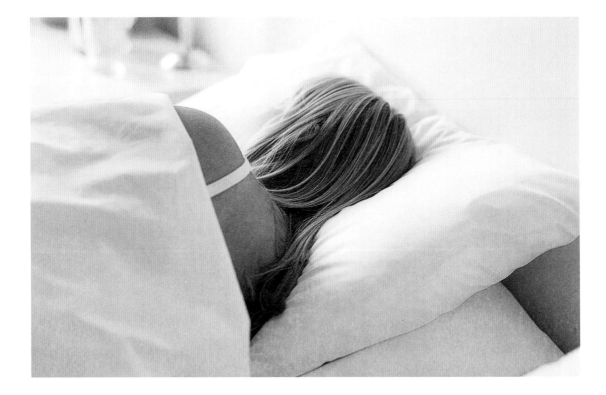

- Moodiness;
- Difficulty concentrating and impaired cognitive performance;
- Trouble recalling information and solving problems;
- Greater awareness of aches and pains;
- Increased propensity to have accidents;
- In extreme cases, disorientation, hallucinations, and paranoia;
- Maybe worst of all, increased difficulty getting back on a comfortable sleep schedule.

Sleep deprivation has an impact on physical health as well, so much so that people are now calling it the new cigarettes (like sitting in chairs; see Chapter 2).[2] It can cause or contribute to:

- Heart disease
- High blood pressure
- Stroke
- Diabetes
- Breast cancer
- Obesity
- Alzheimer's, Parkinson's, and Huntington's diseases.[3]

Why aren't we getting enough sleep? In part, it's because our circadian rhythms are out of sync.

Balanced rhythm

Human beings are creatures of rhythm—from our heartbeats to the pace of our breaths to our sleep cycles—and we should be sleeping when it's dark and waking to the light. These repeating patterns are the ticking of our circadian clock (from the Latin *circa*, meaning about, and *dies*, day). Light is the primary and strongest environmental time cue that calibrates the body's internal clock to pretty much a twenty-four-hour cycle. When our circadian rhythm is out of kilter, so are we, and it's like walking around with permanent jet lag. To optimize our levels of melatonin, the hormone our brain produces at night and that regulates this body clock, we need to be awake when it's light and asleep when it's dark. Exposure to light before bedtime may reduce our sleep quality by suppressing the production of melatonin.

Staying as close as possible to the natural cycles of darkness and light—which usually means going to bed around 10 p.m. and getting up near sunrise—helps to keep our circadian rhythms balanced and can help to diminish insomnia. This is especially important as we get older, since it's been shown that aging results in a significant reduction in daylight sensitivity in the part of the brain that controls circadian rhythms.

There are other things you can do to help yourself sleep better:

- Eat at regular times, and not within three hours of bedtime;
- Get a good dose of sunlight. We know from earlier chapters how healing a sunny window view can be, especially when we're recovering from illness;
- Avoid using electronics or getting too much artificial light in the late evening, and keep electronic devices out of your bedroom if possible.

Chrono-medicine

The current Western research into chrono-medicine or chrono-therapy is fascinating, and so are its parallels to Chinese medicine. It is an approach that involves timing the dosage of medications to minimize their side effects while maximizing their effectiveness, and it is especially powerful when linked to our circadian clock. The researcher Chi Van Dang, scientific director of Ludwig Cancer Research, and many of his fellow cancer researchers are exploring the ways circadian rhythms correlate with the development of tumors. They are also experimenting to find out what impact the timing of doses has on their effectiveness, and finding ways to reset patients' circadian clocks.[4]

The implications for cancer treatment are staggering, and very important, but this technique can also be applied to other medications, such as analgesics, and to supplements. You could experiment with a modified form of chrono-medicine yourself. Try taking your vitamins or pain or allergy medication at different times of the day. Do you notice a particular time when it seems more effective?

Lightening up

As we've seen in previous chapters (especially 1 and 7), daylight matters a lot—almost as much as sleep. We can't all live in Los Angeles or Athens, and those of us in areas that receive less sunlight over the year—such as London, Seattle, or Juneau, Alaska—are prone to seasonal affective disorder (SAD), which disturbs our physical and mental health. Dr. Norman Rosenthal was the first to give a name to this form of depression that so many of us experience in winter, brought on by fluctuations in the release of serotonin by the brain.[5] We now know that doing things that will stimulate our brains to produce more melatonin and skin to produce more vitamin D will help with SAD, and we can find other ways to lighten up, too.

Recent studies and patient care at institutions such as the Center for Light Treatment and Biological Rhythms at Columbia University's Medical Center suggest that light therapy may contribute to the treatment of depression, bipolar disorder, Alzheimer's disease, and particularly SAD. Researchers don't yet know exactly how light works, but they believe that exposure to bright, full-spectrum artificial light during the day resets the circadian clock. This helps people with SAD recalibrate their internal clocks, especially in the winter, when mornings are dark and our natural rhythms shift. "Exposure to an artificial bright light in the morning usually improves their moods,"

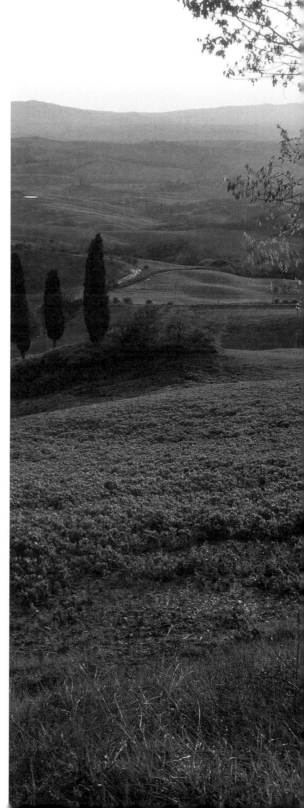

explains Alfred Lewy, a psychiatrist and early researcher into the phenomenon while at the National Institute of Mental Health in the 1980s.[6]

One thing we can do about this is to pay more considered attention to our working and living environments. Increasingly, architects are seeking to maximize opportunities for natural light and darkness in the design of buildings, whether homes, hospitals, or offices. Remember that until the start of the twentieth century our primary source of light was sunlight. Artificial light is a new phenomenon in our biological history.

The nineteenth-century Danish physician Niels Ryberg Finsen was one of the first modern scientists to name and promote light therapy as a medical treatment, and was awarded the Nobel Prize in Medicine in 1903. Since then, there have been many proponents of this basic healing method. Light box therapy is a good option if your lifestyle or job prevents you from connecting to regular day/night rhythms. Most light boxes employ a standard wavelength toward the red end of the color spectrum, usually at an intensity of approximately 10,000 lux, which replicates full daylight but not necessarily direct sun. Opinions as to when and how long to use them vary, so consult a physician or expert before undertaking the treatment.

The dark side of light

The problem is that we don't seem to know when to turn the lights off. LED streetlights were recently installed in my neighborhood, and they are so bright that I can read outdoors at night (probably not a good thing). They seem to be confusing my plants and even changing the growth patterns of the silver maple tree in my yard (definitely not a good thing). These are my unscientific observations, but a growing body of research, including studies from the Max Planck Institute, has shown that most creatures, including humans, need darkness as much as they do light.[7] According to the science writer Dirk Hanson, our twenty-first century overuse of artificial light has disorientated sea turtles, sending them off their natural course, and has interrupted the mating patterns of fireflies.[8] Because of light pollution, one third of the Earth's population can no longer see the Milky Way with the naked eye[9]—and although this is perhaps not a health danger, it is certainly a sad loss of an opportunity to experience beauty and awe.

Hanson puts this into historical perspective, citing late twentieth-century research by William D. Nordhaus, an economist from Yale University, who calculated that in ancient times an average Babylonian would have had to work for 41 hours to afford enough lamp oil to equal an hour's worth of light from a 75-watt bulb. In Colonial America the same amount of light would have required about five hours of work, and nowadays, for the average American using compact fluorescent light bulbs, earning that amount of light would take less than *one second*. This seems a great bargain until you understand its physical and psychological ramifications. Hanson

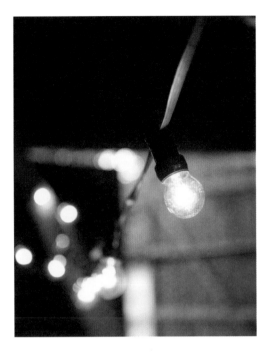

quotes the sleep expert Charles A. Czeisler of Harvard Medical School, who said, "Every time we turn on a light, we are inadvertently taking a drug that affects how we will sleep and how we will be awake the next day."[10]

Recent research has found that preschool-age children exposed to too much light at bedtime showed an 88% reduction in the production of melatonin (the sleep-promoting hormone), because the structure of their young eyes may make them more vulnerable to the impact of bright light.[11] And numerous studies have shown that looking at computers, smartphones, and probably even televisions an hour or so before bed can be disruptive for people of all ages, interfering with our circadian rhythms and causing us to postpone falling asleep naturally, making it more difficult to get up the next morning. The best way to avoid this is to turn off devices and as many lights as you can in the evening, or at least dim the brightness and blue tones on screens.[12]

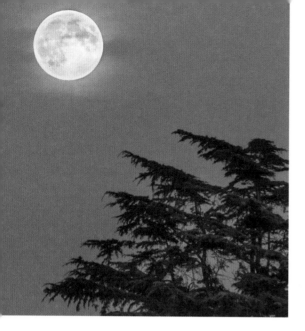

What a little moonlight can do

Moonlight is sunlight reflected from the rocky surface of the moon, and it's about 400,000 times less bright than direct sunlight.[13] Just as the gravitational pull of the moon orchestrates the tides, so it has an effect on the water table and even on the sap in plants. There is no doubt that the moon has an effect on life on Earth, but there is no reliable scientific information on the effect it has on human beings, although there is no lack of anecdotal accounts linking the phases of the moon to hospital admissions, crime rates, animal attacks, and the human reproductive cycle. However, there's a proven connection between moonlight and the reproductive cycles and urgency of marine animals.[14] Going beyond soil, crabs, fish, coral, and other aquatic life, it's not a huge stretch to imagine that mammals, including human beings, could be affected as well.

We have been captivated and charmed by, woven myths around, and even worshipped the moon for as long as we've been on this planet, and maybe that comes back to circadian rhythms and sleep. Before electric light, the moon was our primary nocturnal source of light, and in the present day, as the science writer Claire Asher explains in her blog *Curious Meerkat*,

Research has suggested that sleep quality might vary on a lunar cycle even in the absence of the light stimulus that normally accompanies it. In 2013 a study published in *Current Biology* showed a correlation between sleep quality and the lunar cycle in the laboratory—even in the absence of normal light cues, sleeping people showed variation in their EEG delta activity [the electrical activity of healthy brains, which diminishes with age] during REM sleep [rapid eye-movement sleep, the shallower phase that occurs several times in a night] in line with the lunar cycle. At the full moon, subjects took on average 5 minutes longer to fall asleep, tended to sleep for 20 minutes less and experienced less deep sleep as measured by delta activity during REM sleep. Two other studies have supported these findings, and showed that cortical reactivity, a measure of how deep you are sleeping, is higher at the full moon. People also reported feeling more tired when they awoke.[15]

Further studies were unable to replicate these findings, but it doesn't seem a far-fetched concept. Test it for yourself and see how your sleep patterns shift with the phases of the moon.

Bringing us back to sleep

In *Waking Up to the Dark*, Strand writes about a fascinating phenomenon called "second sleep":

> During the mid-1990s, sleep researcher Thomas Wehr conducted a National Institutes of Health experiment that he later called an exercise in "archaeology, or human paleobiology." Wehr wanted to find out if modern humans still carried within them the rhythms for a prehistoric mode of sleep. Did prehistoric humans sleep more? Did they sleep differently—or perhaps better?[16]

Wehr set up an experiment whereby his subjects lived for an entire month without any form of artificial light whatsoever—completely removed from streetlights, alarm clocks, and any other electronic devices that directed their wakefulness patterns. For the first three weeks the subjects slept for about an hour more per night, but other than that everything was regular. In the fourth week, however, something shifted: They slept for the same total number of hours, but in two increments—about four hours of deep or "first" sleep, two hours of resting wakefulness, then four hours of "second" sleep.

During those two interim hours, the participants reported an unusual state of mind, an almost meditative sense of serenity and peace. Wehr found that their prolactin levels increased soon after dusk and stayed at twice the previously "normal" level during the entire night. Prolactin, a hormone secreted by the pituitary gland, stimulates milk production and maternal feelings in women and has more than 300 other functions in the human body, including those associated with reproduction, metabolism, and immunity; it also seems to be biologically connected to and stimulated by darkness.[17]

But things get even more interesting: These levels of prolactin, which normally decrease at night, remained constant during the wakeful interim period, in contrast to those of people studied (including nightshift workers) who didn't experience the full cycle of natural light and darkness without electric light and woke in the middle of the night. So, perhaps our bodies are hardwired to meditate, to connect with a deeper state of consciousness?

Strand put it beautifully: "I always felt there was something more basic than religion at the bottom of it all. Something simpler. More universal. More rooted in the Earth and its primal rhythms—like the rising and setting of the sun."[18] Wouldn't this resting wakefulness be a lovely phenomenon to reclaim and make part of our way of being?

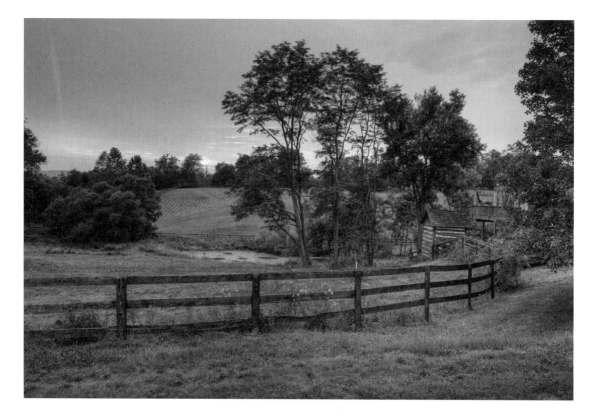

PAY ATTENTION TO THE LIGHT

Try living with as little artificial light as possible:

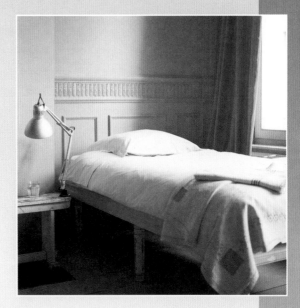

- **When you wake up in the morning,** open the curtains, but wait as long as you can before turning on lights or looking at screens.

- **Limit your computer and smartphone time as much as your job or lifestyle permits,** and take advantage of timers and orange screen settings to filter the artificial blue light.

- **When you walk into a room,** pause and don't automatically turn on the light — think about whether you really need it.

- **Instead of spending your leisure time looking into lights** (watching television, playing video games, or surfing the net), engage in activities where the light is more passive, such as reading, playing board games, cooking or baking, or having a conversation.

- **Block light that seeps into the room where you sleep.** Use heavy shades or lots of potted plants (bonuses: green during the day, and cleaner air) to keep the streetlights out.

- **Be attentive to "second sleep,"** and see if there's a shift in the pattern of your rest.

CHAPTER 10

INNER LANDSCAPE

There is something infinitely healing in the repeated refrains of nature—the assurance that dawn comes after night, and spring after the winter.

Rachel Carson, *The Sense of Wonder* (1965)

BRINGING THE OUTDOORS INTO OUR HOMES AND LIVES

No matter how much we wish to take the green cure and connect with nature out in the world—in neighborhood parks or camping trips, botanic gardens, or even favorite cemeteries—at some point we must all return home. There are ways of incorporating the green cure into our everyday lives that are practical, surprising, and perhaps mystical. How can we sustain this every day, not just as a cure but as a preventative? And how can we help others benefit from something that is healing and accessible to everyone in some capacity?

Biophilic hacks

If we fill our homes with living, growing things, perhaps we can inoculate or at least fortify ourselves against times of difficulty or stress. There's an entire field of study devoted to biophilic design and architecture, applying the German psychologist and sociologist Erich Fromm's term *biophilia*—"the love for humanity and nature, and independence and freedom." The theorist and naturalist E.O. Wilson's biophilia hypothesis proposes that humans have evolved an inherent "urge to affiliate with other forms of life" and to love the beauty of nature. Biophilic design incorporates natural materials and light, vegetation, green views, and other experiences of the natural world into the modern built environment. Feng shui—the Chinese system of creating harmonious environments—operates by similar principles.

If you're in a position to build, renovate, or redecorate your own home, the possibilities are thrilling. Most people are not, but fortunately there are other ways to connect with our biophilia, involving little expenditure of money or effort.

PLANT THERAPY

As we know from Dr. Ulrich's study (see page 12) and many others, there's a science behind why we bring plants and bouquets to people when they're sick or grieving. Even just looking at flowers can make us feel better, and there can be a preventative aspect, too. I made suggestions about houseplants, cut flowers, and greenery in earlier chapters, such as vases of tree branches or stored herbs, but it's not just psychological health that can get a boost—we can improve our physical health, as well.

Living, potted plants can help to purify the air even if you're living on a space station! In the 1980s NASA did a lot of research to determine which ones could remove contaminants, such as benzene, formaldehyde, and ammonia, from the air, and found that the very best ones for the job are peace lilies and chrysanthemums.[1] Unfortunately, both these are toxic to dogs or cats, so in your own home you might want to choose non-toxic plants that still have air-filtering capabilities:[2]

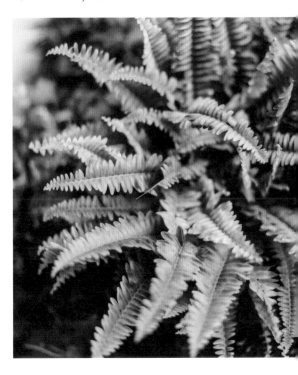

- Date and bamboo palms;
- Boston and Kimberley ferns;
- Spider plants;
- Barberton daisies.

CONSIDER A TERRARIUM

Another way to bring nature into the home is by creating a terrarium. In her essay "Biophilia at My Bedside," Elisabeth Tova Bailey, the author of *The Sounds of a Wild Snail Eating* (2010), wrote of a time when she was confined to bed by a mysterious illness that affected her mitochondrial function and immune system, and she longed for the hikes and time in nature that she could no longer enjoy: "During one of my bedridden years, a terrarium made by a relative became a welcome oasis for my mind. Its small green world distracted me from the intolerable symptoms of illness and the myriad worries of my disabled life." She spent hours entranced by the moss, the spiders, a snail, the unfurling of a fern frond: "Terrariums have gotten me through the coldest winters and the worst stretches of illness; they hold the promise of spring and the hope of convalescence ... a microcosm that contains all of life from birth to death: the challenges, intricacies, and mysteries."[3]

How to create a simple terrarium

- Find a glass container—a large mason jar, a deep wide vase, an abandoned fish tank, or something specially sold for terrariums.
- Spread pebbles or small stones in the bottom of the container, in a layer thick enough that water can drain through (rather like you'd use at the bottom of a flowerpot).
- To stop bacteria from growing in your terrarium, add a thin layer of activated charcoal, which is available inexpensively at pet stores or garden centers.

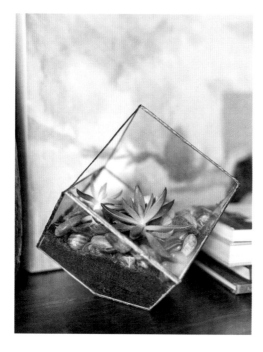

- Top with a layer of potting soil gauged toward the types of plant you'll be using—sandier for succulents, moister for ferns. If in doubt, use a good-quality general-purpose potting medium.
- The plants can be as elaborate or as simple as you like but should have similar light and moisture requirements. Perhaps root cuttings from plants that you already have on hand, or experiment with things like succulents or moss.
- Water about once a week, but do not overwater (keep the soil moist, not waterlogged), and make sure your terrarium gets the right amount of sunlight for the types of plant you've chosen.
- If you have small children or are prone to rescuing creatures, a spider could find a happy home in your terrarium as well.
- If you're feeling ambitious, an aquarium will have many of the same benefits and delights as a terrarium, and aquatic plants are fascinating. However, this would require more expense and more time to maintain.

TOUCHING WOOD

Bringing the green cure into our homes can be simpler and involve even less maintenance than keeping houseplants or making a terrarium. Handling or simply touching objects from nature can bring its own healing. My husband keeps little bits of nature—an acorn, a favorite piece of driftwood, a smooth stone—on his desk, and fidgets with them when he's thinking or creating. It turns out he's onto something. According to a study of the effect of touching wood compared to artificial materials such as metal or plastic, by Chorong Song and her associates of Chiba University's Center for Environment, Health, and Field Sciences in Japan, handling wood resulted in changes to systolic blood pressure, an indicator of decreased physiological stress. Even looking at wood in a home—beams or panels in a living room, for example—had a beneficial effect on blood pressure and pulse rate.[4]

Although we cannot all live in traditional Japanese wood and tatami homes, we can be conscious of the materials we come into contact with during the course of our everyday lives. You might want to choose a wooden chair over a metal or plastic one, and perhaps keep an acorn or other tiny treasure from nature nearby.

TECHNOLOGY AS FRENEMY

Turn it off! We've been conditioned to turn on the light when we enter a room, and close the car windows and switch on the air conditioner when we go for a drive. Sometimes these actions are necessary, but how often are they not? What happens when we enjoy the natural light streaming in at the window and maybe even appreciate an orange sunset that we might have otherwise missed? What happens when we drive through the countryside with the car windows down and catch a breeze or a bit of birdsong? Try it and find out!

Of course, technology is not always the enemy—I for one am devoted to movies on demand, the immediacy of e-books, and the remarkable efficiency of an Internet search—and it can bring more than ease of access. In 2017, studies for the BBC into watching natural history television content found that it can inspire "real happiness" and positive emotional change. Apropos of Wilson's "biophilia" hypothesis, the researchers found that nature immersion, even in the form of still images or video footage, triggers a constellation of responses affecting an individual's emotions, thought patterns, and physiology that enables goal-directed and adaptive actions (such as, in an evolutionary context, focusing on finding food or collaborating on building shelter),[5] hearkening back to Dr. Ulrich's research. It follows that listening to recordings of natural sounds would have a similar result.

Just as a smartphone can be a distraction and take us out of nature and the present moment, so too can it help us to connect with nature. There are apps with real-time stargazing and moon-phase maps that can connect you to the beauty and awe of the night sky. There are others that use facial-recognition techniques to identify plants, trees, and even mushrooms, so that you can learn more about the greenery you pass each day. Go online and search for your favorite botanic garden, planetarium, or natural history museum to find out what they recommend.

Sharing the green cure with others

The American forest ecologist Nalini Nadkarni, a professor of biology at the University of Utah, has made a bold and fascinating point about hospitals. She likens them to prisons, because the "inmates" of both are in situations rife with "extreme stress and anxiety, as their activities and fate are no longer under their own control. Interior spaces are stark and sterile—for punitive and security reasons for prisoners; for health reasons for patients."[6]

In 2004, Nadkarni created the "Moss-in-Prisons" project, which combined tending and observing moss with participating in a conservation undertaking that had an impact beyond the prison walls. She found that it improved social interaction among the inmates and gave them a sense of purpose and meaning as they did something that had value for the wider world.[7] The work she did with prisoners, her "nature intervention," lowered stress and irritability, decreased violence, and fostered a "sense of calmness."[8] Nadkarni sees practicing natural history—and the love that grows out of that action—as a critical thread in the tapestry that makes up our world, an entity that is complex, connected, useful, strong, fragile, and beautiful. Who could disagree? It's a reminder to us all not to forget about the people who might be out of sight, or those who are living in confined or limited situations—not just prisons but places such as nursing homes or assisted living facilities.

WHAT WE CAN DO

As we learn more about the green cure and insights like Nadkarni's, it is only natural to want to share it with others. That might involve something as simple as picking up trash on your way home from work, adopting and tending a street tree, or tossing flower-seed "bombs" into a vacant lot. It might involve helping children to develop an appreciation

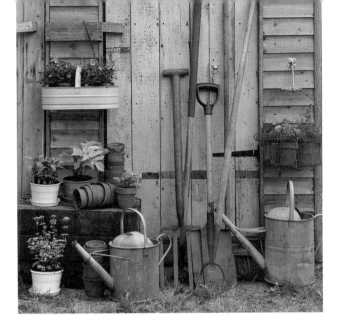

for nature, or just limiting their screen time and giving them more opportunities to play in the mud. It might mean organizing more ways for them to conduct "fieldwork" in botany, geology, astronomy, and other non-classroom learning through programs at school or at afterschool programs.

Sharing the green cure could be more ambitious, such as by making sure older family members and friends have the chance to be in nature by bringing them plants and helping them to tend them. Or better yet, help them to get outdoors. We know from Chapter 5 that gardening and spending time outdoors regularly has benefits for the elderly, and recently a study by the Barcelona Institute for Global Health that followed 6,500 people in the United Kingdom over ten years found that living in a place with natural surroundings may help to prevent cognitive decline in elderly people.[9] The research found that older people who lived in greener neighborhoods tended to lose cognitive function at a slower rate than those who lived where there was less verdure. (Interestingly, there was a stronger impact for women than for men.)

Think about how you can apply these findings to an elderly parent or neighbor. Moving to a new home may not be an option, but planting— especially spots that can be seen from a porch or through a window—might be. You could spend a little more time together, taking your favorite senior citizen for a walk to the local farmers' market instead of picking up groceries for them or driving them to the supermarket. Or, if mobility is a problem for them, even playing them nature videos or sound recordings could help.

SKY GAZING

I started this book looking out the window, so I thought it would be nice
to come full circle and end it the same way. Esteemed American Buddhist
meditation teacher Lama Surya Das shares a sky-gazing meditation that can
be done by anyone at any time—a lovely way to connect and interconnect
with nature. It can promote healing on many levels—meditation fosters basic
relaxation, improved concentration, slowed heart rate, and more—and fill us
with a sense of awe.

Seated with a view of sky or clouds,
Or even just a leaf from a beloved tree,
Close your eyes.
Inhale deeply, and exhale fully,
Letting totally go.
Now do it again, twice more.
(Three is the magic number.)
Let go, let it all come and go;
Let it be.
Just be,
As you are.
Rest naturally and at ease
In your body and mind, heart and soul,
And enjoy the natural state—
or whatever state you seem to be in.
Let body and mind settle in its own place,
Its own way,
Its own time,
As it is.
Natural breath and energy,
Natural flow,
Let it go,

Free from interference, evaluation, or manipulation …
and enjoy the joy
of natural meditation.
Don't be deceived or seduced by momentary
thoughts and experiences.
Allow all experiences to pass freely, like clouds
In a vast, open sky.
Simply Observe, Allow, and Accept.
Embrace and surrender.
Letting go means letting come and go,
letting be.
This is the essence of inner freedom
and autonomy
within interconnection.
Be still
and know
all is well.
All is as it must be, right
here, right now —
this very moment, the only moment;
this very breath, as if the only breath.
Don't let attention stray elsewhere.
Nothing to figure out, understand,
Achieve, track, or remember.
No need to fabricate or contrive;
No need to even meditate.
Simply present, undistracted, at home
And at ease
In the natural state
Of natural perfection,
let awareness unfurl
its myriad colors.
We are within nature, just as nature is within us. We are it and it is us.[10]

ENDNOTES

Introduction

1 Erich Fromm, *The Anatomy of Human Destructiveness* (H. Holt, 1992).

2 Edward Osborne Wilson, *Biophilia* (Harvard University Press, 1984).

3 Richard Louv, *Vitamin N* (Atlantic Books, 2017).

4 Aaron Antonovsky, "A Somewhat Personal Odyssey in Studying the Stress Process," *Stress Medicine*, 6/2 (1990), pp. 71–80.

5 Rick Hanson, *Hardwiring Happiness* (Harmony Books, 2016), p. 12.

6 L.E. Carlson et al., "Mindfulness-based Cancer Recovery and Supportive-expressive Therapy Maintain Telomere Length Relative to Controls in Distressed Breast Cancer Survivors," *Cancer*, 121/3 (February 2015), pp. 476–84, www.ncbi.nlm.nih.gov/pubmed/25367403.

Chapter 1: Fresh Air

1 Roger S. Ulrich, "View Through a Window May Influence Recovery from Surgery," *Science*, 224/4647 (April 27, 1984), pp. 420–1.

2 Ruth Kjærsti Raanaas et al., "Health Benefits of a View of Nature Through the Window: A Quasi-Experimental Study of Patients in a Residential Rehabilitation Center," *Clinical Rehabilitation*, 26/1 (2012), pp. 21–32, www.ncbi.nlm.nih.gov/pubmed/21856720.

3 Cecily Maller et al., "Healthy Nature Healthy People: 'Contact with Nature' as an Upstream Health Promotion Intervention for Populations," *Health Promotion International*, 21/1 (March 1, 2006), pp. 45–54, academic.oup.com/heapro/article/21/1/45/646436.

4 Quoted in Patty Wellborn, "Science Confirms You Should Stop and Smell the Roses," UBC Okanagan News, November 2, 2017, www.news.ok.ubc.ca/2017/11/02/science-confirms-you-should-stop-and-smell-the-roses.

5 Christopher Bergland, "Exposure to Natural Light Improves Workplace Performance," *Psychology Today* blog, June 5, 2013, www.psychologytoday.com/us/blog/the-athletes-way/201306/exposure-natural-light-improves-workplace-performance.

6 J.R. Minkel, "A Breath of Fresh Air: To Fight Tuberculosis, Open a Window," *Scientific American*, February 26, 2007, www.scientificamerican.com/article/a-breath-of-fresh-air-to.

7 Quoted in Robin Finn, "Mold, Come Out with Your Hands Up," *New York Times*, May 3, 2013, www.nytimes.com/2013/05/05/realestate/bill-sothern-remediates-mold-and-other-hazards.html.

8 Carolyn Crist, "Open Windows and Doors Can Improve Sleep Quality," *Reuters*, December 7, 2017, www.reuters.com/article/us-health-sleep/open-windows-and-doors-can-improve-sleep-quality-idUSKBN1E12DK.

9 Jill Neimark, "Extreme Chemical Sensitivity Makes Sufferers Allergic to Life," *Discover*, December 11, 2013, www.discovermagazine.com/2013/nov/13-allergic-life.

10 Petter Erik Leirhaug, "The Role of *Friluftsliv* in Henrik Ibsen's Works," paper delivered at "Henrik Ibsen: The Birth of 'Friluftsliv': A 150-Year International Dialogue Conference Jubilee Celebration," North Troendelag University College, Norway, September 14–19, 2009, www.norwegianjournaloffriluftsliv.com/doc/172010.pdf.

11 Luke (Natural Resources Institute Finland), "The Effects of Nature on Well-Being," www.luke.fi/en/natural-resources/recreational-use-of-nature/the-effects-of-nature-well-being, accessed August 2018.

12 Magdalena M.H.E. van den Berg et al., "Autonomic Nervous System Responses to Viewing Green and Built Settings: Differentiating Between Sympathetic and Parasympathetic Activity," *International Journal of Environmental Research and Public Health*, 12/12 (December 2015), pp. 15,860–74, www.ncbi.nlm.nih.gov/pmc/articles/PMC4690962.

Chapter 2: Take a Walk

1 Howard V. Hong and Edna H. Hong, *The Essential Kierkegaard* (Princeton University Press, 2013), p. 502.

2 "Sitting Is Bad for Your Brain: Not Just Your Metabolism or Heart," *Science Daily*, April 12, 2018, www.sciencedaily.com/releases/2018/04/180412141014.htm.

3 C.E. Matthews et al., "Amount of Time Spent in Sedentary Behaviors and Cause-specific Mortality in US Adults," *American Journal of Clinical Nutrition*, 95/2 (2012), pp. 437–45, www.ncbi.nlm.nih.gov/pubmed/22218159.

4 Jill K. Morris et al., "Aerobic Exercise for Alzheimer's Disease: A Randomized Controlled Pilot Trial," *PLoS One*, 12/2 (February 10, 2017), www.journals.plos.org/plosone/article?id=10.1371/journal.pone.0170547.

5 Byambaa Enkhmaa et al., "Lifestyle Changes: Effect of Diet, Exercise, Functional Food, and Obesity Treatment on Lipids and Lipoproteins," *Endotext*, June 8, 2015, www.ncbi.nlm.nih.gov/books/NBK326737.

6 Esther M. Sternberg, *Healing Spaces* (Belknap Press, 2009).

7 Melissa R. Marselle et al., "Moving beyond Green: Exploring the Relationship of Environment Type and Indicators of Perceived Environmental Quality on Emotional Well-Being following Group Walks," *International Journal of Environmental Research and Public Health*, 12/1 (2015), pp. 106–130.

8 Gregory N. Bratman et al., "Nature Experience Reduces Rumination and Subgenual Prefrontal Cortex Activation," *Proceedings of the National Academy of Sciences of the United States of America*, 112/28 (July 14, 2015), www.pnas.org/content/112/28/8567.

9 Johannes Michalak et al., "How We Walk Affects What We Remember: Gait Modifications Through Biofeedback Change Negative Memory Bias," *Journal of Behavior Therapy and Experimental Psychiatry*, 46 (March 2015), pp. 121–25, quoted in "How To Feel Better By Just Walking Differently," PsyBlog, October 19, 2014, www.spring.org.uk/2014/10/how-to-feel-happy-just-by-walking-differently.php.

10 "Going Outside—Even in the Cold—Improves Memory,

Attention," Michigan News, University of Michigan, December 16, 2008, www.news.umich.edu/going-outsideeven-in-the-coldimproves-memory-attention.

11 Gregory N. Bratman et al., "Nature Experience Reduces Rumination and Subgenual Prefrontal Cortex Activation," *Proceedings of the National Academy of Sciences of the United States of America*, 112/28 (July 14, 2015), www.pnas.org/content/112/28/8567.

12 May Wong, "Stanford Study Finds Walking Improves Creativity," Stanford News, April 24, 2014, https://news.stanford.edu/2014/04/24/walking-vs-sitting-042414.

13 Clark Strand, *Waking Up to the Dark* (Spiegel & Grau, 2015), p. 17.

14 Thich Nhat Hanh, *Present Moment, Wonderful Moment* (Parallax Press, 2002), p. 57.

Chapter 3: Shinrin-yoku

1 Ahmad Hassan et al., "Effects of Walking in Bamboo Forest and City Environments on Brainwave Activity in Young Adults," *Evidence-based Complementary and Alternative Medicine*, 2018, www.hindawi.com/journals/ecam/2018/9653857.

2 "Immerse Yourself in a Forest for Better Health," New York State Department of Environmental Conservation, www.dec.ny.gov/lands/90720.html, accessed August 2018.; Gen Xiang Mao et al., "Additive Benefits of Twice Forest Bathing Trips in Elderly Patients with Chronic Heart Failure," *Biomedical and Environmental Sciences*, 31/2 (February 2018), www.ncbi.nlm.nih.gov/pubmed/29606196.

3 Kyoung Sang Cho et al., "Terpenes from Forests and Human Health," *Toxicology Research*, 33/2 (April 2017), pp. 97–106, www.ncbi.nlm.nih.gov/pubmed/28443180.

4 Quoted in Diane Toomey, "How Listening to Trees Can Help Reveal Nature's Connections," *Yale Environment 360*, August 24, 2017, www.e360.yale.edu/features/how-listening-to-trees-can-help-reveal-natures-connections.

5 Richard Grant, "Do Trees Talk to Each Other?," *Smithsonian*, March 2018, www.smithsonianmag.com/science-nature/the-whispering-trees-180968084.

6 See www.greencitysolutions.de/en/solutions.

7 David G. Haskell, *The Songs of Trees* (Viking Press, 2017), p. vii.

Chapter 4: Delightful Dirt

1 M.E. O'Brien et al., "SRL172 (Killed Mycobacterium vaccae) in Addition to Standard Chemotherapy Improves Quality of Life Without Affecting Survival, in Patients with Advanced Non-small-cell Lung Cancer: Phase III Results," *Annals of Oncology*, 15/6 (June 2004), pp. 906–14, www.ncbi.nlm.nih.gov/pubmed/15151947.

2 Jenni Laidman, "Microbes Rule Your Health—and Further Prove that Kids Should Eat Dirt," *Chicago Tribune*, October 13, 2017, www.chicagotribune.com/lifestyles/health/sc-hlth-microbiome-1018-story.html.

3 Linda Chen, "The Old and Mysterious Practice of Eating Dirt, Revealed," *NPR*, April 2, 2014, www.npr.org/sections/thesalt/2014/04/02/297881388/the-old-and-mysterious-practice-of-eating-dirt-revealed.

4 Lisa Elaine Held, "5 Foods That Have More Potassium Than a Banana," *Well+Good*, September 15, 2011, www.wellandgood.com/good-advice/5-foods-that-have-more-potassium-than-a-banana.

5 Elise Alvaro et al., "Composition and Metabolism of the Intestinal Microbiota in Consumers and Non-consumers of Yogurt," *British Journal of Nutrition*, 97/1 (January 2007), www.ncbi.nlm.nih.gov/pubmed/17217568.

6 Ruairi Robertson, "10 Ways to Improve Your Gut Bacteria, Based on Science," *Healthline*, November 18, 2016, www.healthline.com/nutrition/improve-gut-bacteria#section5.

7 Ibid.

8 James L. Oschman et al., "The Effects of Grounding (Earthing) on Inflammation, the Immune Response, Wound Healing, and Prevention and Treatment of Chronic Inflammatory and Autoimmune Diseases," *Journal of Inflammation Research*, 8 (March 24, 2015), pp. 83–96, www.ncbi.nlm.nih.gov/pmc/articles/PMC4378297.

9 Antygona Chadzopulu et al., "The Therapeutic Effects of Mud," *Progressive Health Sciences*, 1/2 (2011), www.nymedicalcare.com/Docs/mud.pdf.

10 Hagit Matz, Edith Orion, and Ronni Wolf, "Balneotherapy in Dermatology," *Dermatologic Therapy*, 16 (2003), pp. 132–40, www.sld.cu/galerias/pdf/sitios/rehabilitacion-bal/matzh_et_al.pdf.

Chapter 5: Plant Therapy

1 Mihaly Csikszentmihalyi, *Flow* (HarperCollins, 1991).

2 Gardening Matters, "Multiple Benefits of Community Gardening," 2012, www.gardeningmatters.org/sites/default/files/Multiple%20Benefits_2012.pdf.

3 "Quotes by Hildegard of Bingen," *Healthy Hildegard*, www.healthyhildegard.com/hildegard-bingen-quotes, accessed August 2018.

4 Agnes E. Van Den Berg and Mariëtte H. Custers, "Gardening Promotes Neuroendocrine and Affective Restoration from Stress," *Journal of Health Psychology*, 16/1 (January 2011), pp. 3–11, www.ncbi.nlm.nih.gov/pubmed/20522508.

5 Anne Harding, "Why Gardening is Good for Your Health," *CNN*, July 8, 2011, www.cnn.com/2011/HEALTH/07/08/why.gardening.good/index.html.

6 Elizabeth A. Barley et al., "Primary-care Based Participatory Rehabilitation: Users' Views of a Horticultural and Arts Project," *British Journal of General Practice*, 62/595 (January 30, 2012), pp. e127–e134, www.ncbi.nlm.nih.gov/pmc/articles/PMC3268492.

7 Miho Igarashi et al., "Physiological and Psychological Effects of Viewing a Kiwifruit (*Actinidia deliciosa* 'Hayward') Orchard Landscape in Summer in Japan," *International Journal of Environmental Research and Public Health*, 12/6 (June 2015), pp. 6657–68, www.ncbi.nlm.nih.gov/pmc/articles/PMC4483722.

8 American Horticultural Therapy Association, "Horticultural Therapy," www.ahta.org/horticultural-therapy, accessed August 2018.

9 Jane S. Hirschi, *Ripe for Change: Garden-based Learning in Schools* (Harvard Education Press, 2015).

10 "Being Raised in Greener Neighborhoods May Have Beneficial Effects on Brain Development," *Neuroscience News*, February 23, 2018, www.neurosciencenews.com/brain-development-green-environment-8551.

11 Tyra A. Olstad, *Zen of the Plains: Experiencing Wild Western Places* (University of North Texas Press, 2014), p. 235.

12 CIRIA, "Psychological," www.opengreenspace.com/opportunities-and-challenges/health/psychological, accessed August 2018.

13 "Why Green Spaces Are Good for Gray Matter," *Neuroscience News*, April 10, 2017, www.neurosciencenews.com/green-spaces-neurobiology-6376.

14 Robin Wall Kimmerer, *Braiding Sweetgrass* (Milkweed Editions, 2014), p. 10.

15 Diana Beresford-Kroeger, *The Sweetness of a Simple Life* (Vintage Canada, 2015) p. 77.

Chapter 6: The Sense of Nature

1 Peter Aspinall et al., "The Urban Brain: Analysing Outdoor Physical Activity with Mobile EEG," *British Journal of Sports Medicine*, 49/4 (February 2015), pp. 272–76, www.ncbi.nlm.nih.gov/pubmed/23467965; Chris Neale et al., 'The Ageing Urban Brain: Analyzing Outdoor Physical Activity Using the Emotiv Affectiv Suite in Older People," *Journal of Urban Health*, 94/6 (December 2017), pp. 869–80, https://link.springer.com/article/10.1007/s11524-017-0191-9.

2 R. S. Ulrich, "View Through a Window May Influence Recovery from Surgery," *Science*, 224/4647 (April 27, 1984), pp. 420–421.

3 Sternberg, *Healing Spaces*.

4 Edward A. Vessel and Irving Biedermann, "Why Do We Prefer Looking at Some Scenes Rather than Others?," talk presented at OPAM, a conference on Object Perception and Memory, 2001, www.cns.nyu.edu/~vessel/pubs/Vessel_OPAM2001_print.pdf.

5 Sarah Laxmi Chellappa et al., "Photic Memory for Executive Brain Responses," *Proceedings of the National Academy of Sciences*, 111/16 (April 22, 2014): pp. 6087–091, www.pnas.org/content/111/16/6087.

6 Quoted in Wallace J. Nicholls, *Blue Mind* (Little, Brown, 2014), p. 89.

7 Chorong Song, Harumi Ikei, and Yoshifumi Miyazaki, "Physiological Effects of Nature Therapy: A Review of the Research in Japan," *International Journal of Environmental Research and Public Health*, 13/8 (August 2016), p. 781, www.ncbi.nlm.nih.gov/pmc/articles/PMC4997467.

8 Sarah Laxmi Chellappa et al., "Photic Memory for Executive Brain Responses," *Proceedings of the National Academy of Sciences*, 111/16 (April 22, 2014): pp. 6087–091, www.pnas.org/content/111/16/6087.

9 Qing Li, *Forest Bathing* (Penguin, 2018).

10 Richard Taylor, "Fractal Patterns in Nature and Art Are Aesthetically Pleasing and Stress-reducing," *The Conversation*, March 31, 2017, www.theconversation.com/fractal-patterns-in-nature-and-art-are-aesthetically-pleasing-and-stress-reducing-73255.

11 Andrew J. Johnson, "Cognitive Facilitation Following Intentional Odor Exposure," *Sensors*, 11/5 (2011), pp. 5469–88, www.ncbi.nlm.nih.gov/pubmed/22163909.

12 Tapanee Hongratanaworakit, "Relaxing Effect of Rose Oil on Humans," *Natural Product Communications*, 4/2 (February 2009), pp. 291–96, www.ncbi.nlm.nih.gov/pubmed/19370942.

13 Lyz Cooper, *#What Is Sound Healing?* (Watkins, 2016).

14 Cassandra D. Gould van Praag et al., "Mind-wandering and Alterations to Default Mode Network Connectivity When Listening to Naturalistic Versus Artificial Sounds," *Scientific Reports*, 7 (2017), www.nature.com/articles/srep45273.

15 "How the Sounds of Nature Help Us to Relax," *Neuroscience News*, March 30, 2017, www.neurosciencenews.com/nature-sound-relaxation-6311.

16 Jesper J. Alvarsson, Stefan Wiens, and Mats E. Nilsson, "Stress Recovery During Exposure to Nature Sound and Environmental Noise," *International Journal of Environmental Research and Public Health*, 7/3 (March 2010), pp. 1036–46, www.ncbi.nlm.nih.gov/pmc/articles/PMC2872309.

17 Denise Winterman, "The Surprising Uses for Birdsong," *BBC News*, May 8, 2013, www.bbc.com/news/magazine-22298779.

18 George Prochnik, *In Pursuit of Silence* (Doubleday Books, 2010), p. 237.

19 "Raisin Meditation," https://ggia.berkeley.edu/practice/raisin_meditation#

Chapter 7: From Thunderstorms to Desert Heat

1 Peter Wohlleben, *The Weather Detective* (Rider, 2018).

2 "How Our Bodies React to Weather," *Japan Today*, May 31, 2017, www.japantoday.com/category/features/kuchikomi/how-our-bodies-react-to-weather.

3 Patrick Baylis et al., "Weather Impacts Expressed Sentiment," *PLoS One*, 13/4 (April 25, 2018), www.journals.plos.org/plosone/article?id=10.1371/journal.pone.0195750.

4 Megan Ware, "What Are the Health Benefits of Vitamin D?," *Medical News Today*, November 13, 2017, www.medicalnewstoday.com/articles/161618.php.

5 Hafid Ait-Oufella and Andrew P. Sage, "The Sunlight: A New Immunomodulatory Approach of Atherosclerosis," *Arteriosclerosis, Thrombosis, and Vascular Biology*, 37 (2017), pp. 7–9, http://atvb.ahajournals.org/content/37/1/7.

6 Sian Geldenhuys et al., "Ultraviolet Radiation Suppresses Obesity and Symptoms of Metabolic Syndrome Independently of Vitamin D in Mice Fed a High-fat Diet," *Diabetes*, 63/11 (November 2014), pp. 3759–69, www.ncbi.nlm.nih.gov/pubmed/25342734.

7 Shelley Gorman et al., "Can Skin Exposure to Sunlight Prevent Liver Inflammation?," *Nutrients*, 7/5 (May 2015), pp. 3219–3239, www.ncbi.nlm.nih.gov/pmc/articles/PMC4446748.

8 "Niels Ryberg Finsen: Biographical," Nobel Prize website, from *Nobel Lectures, Physiology or Medicine 1901–1921* (Elsevier, 1967), www.nobelprize.org/nobel_prizes/medicine/laureates/1903/finsen-bio.html.

9 Kleyton de Carvalho Mesquita, Ana Carolina de Souza Machado Igreja, and Izelda Maria Carvalho Costa, "Atopic Dermatitis and Vitamin D: Facts and Controversies," *Anais Brasileiros de Dermatologia*, 88/6 (2013), pp. 945–953, www.ncbi.nlm.nih.gov/pmc/articles/PMC3900346.

10 James Close, "Are Stress Responses to Geomagnetic Storms Mediated by the Cryptochrome Compass System?," *Proceedings of the Royal Society B*, March 14, 2012, http://rspb.royalsocietypublishing.org/content/279/1736/2081.

11 Alex Myles, "Major Solar Storms Causing Anxiety, Fatigue and Powerful Energy Shifts: March 16th–26th," *Elephant Journal*, March 16, 2018, www.elephantjournal.com/2018/03/major-solar-storms-causing-anxiety-fatigue-powerful-energy-shifts-march-16th-26th.

12 Christie Nicholson, "Fact or Fiction? 'Spring Fever' Is a Real Phenomenon," *Scientific American*, March 22, 2007, www.scientificamerican.com/article/fact-or-fiction-spring-fever-is-a-real-phenomenon.

13 "Feeling Flirty? Wait for the Sun to Shine," *Science Daily*, January 28, 2013, www.sciencedaily.com/releases/2013/01/130128081950.htm.

14 Judy Willis, "The Science of Spring: How a Change of Seasons Can Boost Classroom Learning," *Guardian*, April 2, 2015, www.theguardian.com/teacher-network/2015/apr/02/science-spring-how-seasons-classroom-learning.

15 Denise Mann, "Negative Ions Create Positive Vibes," *WebMD*, www.webmd.com/balance/features/negative-ions-create-positive-vibes.

16 Vanessa Perez, Dominik D. Alexander, and William H. Bailey, "Air Ions and Mood Outcomes: A Review and Meta-analysis," *BMC Psychiatry*, 13 (2013), p. 29, www.ncbi.nlm.nih.gov/pmc/articles/PMC3598548.

17 See Dictionary.com, www.dictionary.com/browse/petrichor.

18 Joseph Stromberg, "What Makes Rain Smell so Sweet?," *Smithsonian Magazine*, April 2, 2013, www.smithsonianmag.com/science-nature/what-makes-rain-smell-so-good-13806085.

19 Ibid.

20 John Goodwin, *Weather and the Mind* (Lichtenstein Creative Media, 2001), p. 6.

21 Willis H. Miller, "Santa Ana Winds and Crime," *The Professional Geographer*, 20/1 (January 1968), pp. 23–27, www.onlinelibrary.wiley.com/doi/abs/10.1111/j.0033-0124.1968.00023.x.

22 "Out in the Cold," Harvard Health Letter, January 2010, www.health.harvard.edu/staying-healthy/out-in-the-cold.

23 Marjo Tourula, "The Childcare Practice of Children's Daytime Sleeping Outdoors in the Context of Northern Finnish Winter," *ACTA*, 2011, www.fatherly.com/wp-content/uploads/2015/10/isbn9789514296673.pdf.

24 Meaghan Brown, "The Surprising Benefits of Training in the Heat," *Outside*, July 21, 2016, www.outsideonline.com/2098556/surprising-benefits-training-heat.

25 Tanjaniina Laukkanen et al., "Association Between Sauna Bathing and Fatal Cardiovascular and All-cause Mortality Events," *JAMA Internal Medicine*, 175/4 (April 2015), pp. 542–48, https://jamanetwork.com/journals/jamainternalmedicine/fullarticle/2130724.

26 Mikko Norros, "Bare Facts of the Sauna," *This Is Finland*, December 2001, www.finland.fi/life-society/bare-facts-of-the-sauna.

Chapter 8: Water Treatment

1 Mircea Eliade, *Patterns in Comparative Religion* (1958), p. 194.

2 Rafi Letzter, "How Long Can a Person Survive Without Water?," *Live Science*, November 29, 2017, www.livescience.com/32320-how-long-can-a-person-survive-without-water.html.

3 Anne Marie Helmenstine, "How Much of Your Body Is Water?," *ThoughtCo.*, June 1, 2018, www.thoughtco.com/how-much-of-your-body-is-water-609406.

4 "The Water in You," United States Geological Survey, https://water.usgs.gov/edu/propertyyou.html, accessed August 2018.

5 "Drinking More Water Associated with Numerous Dietary Benefits, Study Finds," *Science Daily*, March 1, 2016, www.sciencedaily.com/releases/2016/03/160301174759.htm.

6 "A Guide to Drinking Water Treatment and Sanitation for Backcountry Use and Travel," Centers for Disease Control and Prevention, www.cdc.gov/healthywater/drinking/travel/backcountry_water_treatment.html, accessed August 2018.

7 "Bottled Water Contains More Bacteria than Tap Water," *The Telegraph*, May 25, 2010, www.telegraph.co.uk/news/health/news/7763038/bottled-water-contains-more-bacteria-than-tap-water.html.

8 "270 Million Visits Made to English Coastlines Each Year," *Science Daily*, April 5, 2018, www.sciencedaily.com/releases/2018/04/180405120359.htm.

9 Wallace J. Nichols, *Blue Mind* (Little, Brown 2014), p. 155.

10 Benedict W. Wheeler et al., "Does Living by the Coast Improve Health and Wellbeing?," *Health & Place*, 18/5 (September 2012), pp. 1198–1201, www.doi.org/10.1016/j.healthplace.2012.06.015.

11 Mathew P. White et al., "The Effects of Exercising in Different Natural Environments on Psycho-Physiological Outcomes in Post-Menopausal Women: A Simulation Study," *International Journal of Environmental Research and Public Health*, 12 (2015), pp. 11,929–53, https://pdfs.semanticscholar.org/45f2/095769b7fdf1552d2ca523c35b96dffdc17c.pdf.

12 Ibid.

13 "Percentage of Total Population Living in Coastal Areas," United Nations, www.un.org/esa/sustdev/natlinfo/indicators/methodology_sheets/oceans_seas_coasts/pop_coastal_areas.pdf.

14 Deborah Cracknell et al., "Marine Biota and Psychological Well-Being: A Preliminary Examination of Dose-Response Effects in an Aquarium Setting," *Environment and Behavior*, 48/10 (December 2016), pp. 1242–69, http://journals.sagepub.com/doi/abs/10.1177/0013916515597512.

15 Quoted in Mark Kinver, "Aquariums 'Deliver Significant Health Benefits,'" *BBC News*, July 30, 2015, www.bbc.com/news/science-environment-33716589.

16 Eun-Sun Hwang, Kyung-Nam Ki, and Ha-Yull Chang, "Proximate Composition, Amino Acid, Mineral, and Heavy Metal Content of Dried Laver," *Preventive Nutrition and Food Science*, 18/2 (June 2013), pp. 139–44, www.ncbi.nlm.nih.gov/pmc/articles/PMC3892503.

17 "Where to Harvest Seaweed and How to Eat It," Forage SF, October 14, 2015, www.foragesf.com/blog/2015/10/14/where-to-harvest-seaweed-and-how-to-eat-it.

18 Kazuko Kito and Keiko Suzuki, "Research on the Effect of the Foot Bath and Foot Massage on Residual Schizophrenia Patients," *Archives of Psychiatric Nursing*, 30/3 (June 2016), pp. 375–81, www.sciencedirect.com/science/article/pii/S0883941716000030.

19 Ibid.

20 Tom B. Mole and Pieter Mackeith, "Cold Forced Open-water Swimming: A Natural Intervention to Improve Post-operative Pain and Mobilisation Outcomes?," *BMJ*, 2018, www.sciencedaily.com/releases/2018/02/180212190941.htm.

21 "A Hot Bath Has Benefits Similar to Exercise," *The Conversation*, March 20, 2017, www.theconversation.com/a-hot-bath-has-benefits-similar-to-exercise-74600.

22 François Bieuzen, Chris M. Bleakley, and Joseph Thomas Costello, "Contrast Water Therapy and Exercise-induced Muscle Damage: A Systematic Review and Meta-analysis," *PLoS One*, 8/4 (April 2013), http://journals.plos.org/plosone/article?id=10.1371/journal.pone.0062356.

23 Benoît Dugué and Esa Leppänen, "Adaptation Related to Cytokines in Man: Effects of Regular Swimming in Ice-cold Water," *Clinical Physiology*, 20/2 (March 2000), pp. 114–21, www.ncbi.nlm.nih.gov/pubmed/10735978.

24 Ian M. Wilcock, John B. Cronin, and Wayne A. Hing, "Water Immersion: Does It Enhance Recovery from Exercise?," *International Journal of Sports Physiology and Performance*, 1/3 (September 2006), pp. 195–206, www.ncbi.nlm.nih.gov/pubmed/19116434.

25 Carina Grafetstätter et al., "Does Waterfall Aerosol Influence Mucosal Immunity and Chronic Stress? A Randomized Controlled Clinical Trial," *Journal of Physiological Anthropology*, 36/10 (2017), www.ncbi.nlm.nih.gov/pmc/articles/PMC5237191.

26 Quoted in Adam Hadhazy, "Why Does the Sound of Water Help You Sleep?," *Live Science*, January 18, 2016, www.livescience.com/53403-why-sound-of-water-helps-you-sleep.html.

Chapter 9: Circadian Rhythms

1 "Sleep Scientist Warns Against Walking Through Life 'in an Underslept State,'" *Daily Good*, October 16, 2017, www.dailygood.org/more.php?n=7686.

2 "Sleep Loss Linked to Nighttime Snacking, Junk Food Cravings, Obesity, Diabetes," *Science Daily*, June 1, 2018, www.sciencedaily.com/releases/2018/06/180601171900.htm; Camille Peri, "10 Things to Hate About Sleep Loss," *WebMD*, www.webmd.com/sleep-disorders/features/10-results-sleep-loss.

3 "Antioxidant Benefits of Sleep," *Neuroscience News*, July 13, 2018, www.neurosciencenews.com/sleep-antioxidant-9566.

4 Elie Dolgin, "How to Ruin Cancer's Day," *Knowable*, May 1, 2018, www.knowablemagazine.org/article/health-disease/2018/how-ruin-cancers-day.

5 "What is Seasonal Affective Disorder?," www.normanrosenthal.com/seasonal-affective-disorder.

6 Quoted in Katherine Hobson, "Take Light, Not Drugs," *Nautilus*, March 20, 2014, www.nautil.us/issue/11/light/take-light-not-drugs.

7 Rebecca Boyle, "The End of Night," *Aeon*, April 1, 2014, aeon.co/essays/we-can-t-thrive-in-a-world-without-darkness.

8 Dirk Hanson, "Drowning in Light," *Nautilus*, March 6, 2014, nautil.us/issue/11/light/drowning-in-light.

9 Fabio Falchi et al., "The New World Atlas of Artificial Night Sky Brightness," *Science Advances*, 2/6 (June 2016), e1600377, advances.sciencemag.org/content/2/6/e1600377.full.

10 Jeanne F. Duffy and Charles A. Czeisler, "Effect of Light on Human Circadian Physiology," *Sleep Medicine Clinics*, 4 (2009), pp. 165–77, quoted in Hanson, "Drowning in Light."

11 NOAA, "One-Third of Humanity Can't See the Milky Way," Astronomy.com, June 13, 2016, www.astronomy.com/news/2016/06/one-third-of-humanity-cant-see-the-milky-way.

12 Debra Bradley Ruder, "Circadian Rhythms and the Brain," *On the Brain*, https://neuro.hms.harvard.edu/harvard-mahoney-neuroscience-institute/brain-newsletter/and-brain-series/circadian-rhythms-and-brain, accessed August 2018.

13 Tony Phillips, "Strange Moonlight," NASA, October 3, 2006, www.nasa.gov/vision/universe/watchtheskies/28sep_strangemoonlight.html

14 Ferris Jabr, "How Moonlight Sets Nature's Rhythms," *Hakai Magazine*, June 21, 2017, www.smithsonianmag.com/science-nature/how-moonlight-sets-natures-rhythms-180963778.

15 Claire Asher, "How the Moon Affects Us," *Curious Meerkat* blog, October 29, 2014, www.curiousmeerkat.co.uk/indepth/moon-affects-us.

16 Strand, *Waking Up to the Dark*, p.8.

17 See www.yourhormones.info/hormones/prolactin.

18 Clark Strand, "Want to Enjoy the Deep, Mystical Sleep of Our Ancestors? Turn Your Lights Off at Dusk," *Washington Post*, May 19, 2015, www.washingtonpost.com/news/inspired-life/wp/2015/05/19/want-to-experience-the-deep-mystical-sleep-of-our-ancestors-turn-your-lights-off-at-dusk.

Chapter 10: Inner Landscape

1 B.C. Wolverton et al., "Foliage Plants for Removing Indoor Air Pollutants from Energy-efficient Homes," *Economic Botany*, 38/2 (1984), pp. 224–28, www.jstor.org/stable/4254614?seq=1#page_scan_tab_contents.

2 en.wikipedia.org/wiki/NASA_Clean_Air_Study.

3 Elisabeth Tova Bailey, "Biophilia at My Bedside," in Thomas Lowe Fleischner, ed., *Nature, Love, Medicine* (Torrey House Press, 2017), Kindle version, location 2106, 62%.

4 Chorong Song, Harumi Ikei, and Yoshifumi Miyazaki, ed. Paul B. Tchounwou, "Physiological Effects of Nature Therapy: A Review of the Research in Japan," *International Journal of Environmental Research and Public Health*, 13/8 (August 2016), p. 781, www.ncbi.nlm.nih.gov/pmc/articles/PMC4997467.

5 Dacher Keltner, Richard Bowman, and Harriet Richards, "Exploring the Emotional State of 'Real Happiness': A Study into the Effects of Watching Natural History Television Content," 2017, https://asset-manager.bbcchannels.com/workspace/uploads/bbcw-real-happiness-white-paper-final-v2-58ac1df7.pdf.

6 Nalini Nadkarni, "Branching Out," in Fleischner, *Nature, Love, Medicine*, Kindle version, location 431, 13%.

7 Ibid.

8 Ibid.

9 "Living in Greener Neighborhoods Is Associated with Slower Cognitive Decline in Elderly," *Science Daily*, July 11, 2018, www.sciencedaily.com/releases/2018/07/180711182741.htm.

10 Lama Surya Das, "Sky Gazing", *Make Me One with Everything* (Sounds True, 2015).

BIBLIOGRAPHY

A

"About Hildegard," *Healthy Hildegard*, July 23, 2018, www.healthyhildegard.com/about-hildegard/page/3

Adams, Kathy, "Native American Mosquito Repellent," *Home Guides*, SF Gate, October 7, 2016, http://homeguides.sfgate.com/native-american-mosquito-repellent-76112.html

Allsup, Kelly, "The Restorative Power of Nature," Pantagraph.com, May 26, 2018, www.pantagraph.com/lifestyles/home-and-garden/allsup-the-restorative-power-of-nature/article_df73d799-11fe-5425-b01c-29e49f1389d4.html

American Horticultural Therapy Association, "Definitions and Positions Paper," June 2017, https://ahta.memberclicks.net/assets/docs/definitions%20and%20positions%20final%206.17.pdf

Antonovsky, Aaron, "A Somewhat Personal Odyssey in Studying the Stress Process," *Stress Medicine*, 6/2 (1990), pp. 71–80

Augustin, Sally, "Open the Windows!," *Psychology Today*, August 24, 2015, www.psychologytoday.com/us/blog/people-places-and-things/201508/open-the-windows

B

Baggaley, Kate, "Even If You Live in a City, You Can Get Health Benefits from Nature," *Popular Science*, June 14, 2018, www.popsci.com/city-health-benefits-nature

Baird, Trina-Marie, "How Did Walking Serve as an Integrative Activity for Wordsworth?," (Department of Religious Studies, Lancaster University, 2008)

Barratt, Sarah, "How Sleeping with Your Window Open Is Better for Your Health, According to New Research," *Country Living*, March 29, 2018, www.countryliving.com/uk/wellbeing/news/a2914/open-window-better-nights-sleep

Beasley, Brett, "Bad Air: Pollution, Sin, and Science Fiction in William Delisle Hay's *The Doom of the Great City* (1880)," *Public Domain Review*, September 30, 2015, www.publicdomainreview.org/2015/09/30/bad-air-pollution-sin-and-science-fiction

Beck, Julie, "Nature Therapy Is a Privilege," *The Atlantic*, June 23, 2017, www.theatlantic.com/health/archive/2017/06/how-to-harness-natures-healing-power/531438

Beresford-Kroeger, Diana, *The Sweetness of a Simple Life* (Vintage, 2013)

Berman, Marc G., et al., "Interacting with Nature Improves Cognition and Affect for Individuals with Depression," *Journal of Affective Disorders*, 140/3 (November 2012), pp. 300–5, www.ncbi.nlm.nih.gov/pubmed/22464936

—, John Jonides, and Stephen Kaplan, "The Cognitive Benefits of Interacting with Nature," *Psychological Science*, 19/12 (December 2008), pp. 1207–12, www.ncbi.nlm.nih.gov/pubmed/19121124

Berto, Rita, "Exposure to Restorative Environments Helps Restore Attentional Capacity," *Journal of Environmental Psychology*, 25/3 (September 2005), pp. 249–59, www.sciencedirect.com/science/article/pii/S0272494405000381

Blanding, Michael, "Garden of Ideas," *MIT News*, March 8, 2018, http://news.mit.edu/2018/garden-ideas-anne-whiston-spirn-multimedia-website-0308

Boeschenstein, Nell, "Why Writers Should Consider the Habits of the Flâneur," *Jane Friedman*, April 25, 2016, www.janefriedman.com/walking

Brooks, Libby, "Outdoor Learning Grows in Scotland as Grasp of Benefits Takes Root," *The Guardian*, April 2, 2018, www.theguardian.com/education/2018/apr/02/forest-schools-grow-in-scotland-as-grasp-of-benefits-takes-root

Burke, Edmund, "Of the Sublime," from *On the Sublime and Beautiful* (Harvard Classics, 1909–14), available at www.bartleby.com/24/2/107.html

Burrows, Sara, "We Lock Our Kids up Longer than We Do Maximum Security Convicts," *Newsweek*, October 27, 2017, www.newsweek.com/we-lock-our-kids-longer-we-do-maximum-security-convicts-694845

C

Capaldi, Colin A., L. Dopko Raelyne, and John M. Zelenski, "The Relationship between Nature Connectedness and Happiness: A Meta-Analysis," *Frontiers in Psychology*, 5 (2014), p. 976, www.ncbi.nlm.nih.gov/pmc/articles/PMC4157607

Charpentier, Feline, "Take It Outside: Why Teenagers Need a Daily Fix of Nature," *Tes*, May 11, 2018, www.tes.com/news/tes-magazine/tes-magazine/take-it-outside-why-teenagers-need-a-daily-fix-nature

Chen, Angela, "How Our Body's Circadian Clocks Affect Our Health beyond Sleep," *The Verge*, June 12, 2018, www.theverge.com/2018/6/12/17453398/sleep-circadian-code-satchin-panda-clock-health-science

Chevalier, Gaétan, et al., "Earthing: Health Implications of Reconnecting the Human Body to the Earth's Surface Electrons," *Journal of Environmental and Public Health*, 2012 (2012), p. 291,541, www.ncbi.nlm.nih.gov/pmc/articles/PMC3265077

Clark, Ed, and Marty Brennan, "Why Light Matters: Designing with Circadian Health in Mind," *Metropolis*, March 16, 2017, www.metropolismag.com/interiors/healthcare-interiors/why-light-matters-designing-with-circadian-health-in-mind

"Cold Open Water Plunge Provides Instant Pain Relief, Case Reports Suggest," *Science Daily*, February 12, 2018, www.sciencedaily.com/releases/2018/02/180212190941.htm

Collins, Belinda Lowenhaupt, "Windows and People: A Literature Survey: A Psychological Reaction to Environments with and without Windows," US Department of Commerce, NBS Building Science

Series, no. 70 (1975), https://nvlpubs.nist.gov/nistpubs/Legacy/BSS/nbsbuildingscience70.pdf

Cullinan, Cormac, "If Nature Had Rights," *Orion Magazine*, January 2008, www.orionmagazine.org/article/if-nature-had-rights

D

Dadvand, Payam, et al., "Lifelong Residential Exposure to Green Space and Attention: A Population-based Prospective Study," *Environmental Health Perspectives*, 125/9 (September 2017), www.ncbi.nlm.nih.gov/pubmed/28934095

Das, Lama Surya, *Make Me One with Everything* (Sounds True, 2015)

Donsbach, Kurt W., and Morton Walker, *Negative Ions* (International Institute of Natural Health Science, 1981)

E

Emerson, Ralph Waldo, *Nature* (1836), available at www.online-literature.com/emerson/nature

"Erich Fromm," *Wikipedia*, https://en.wikipedia.org/wiki/Erich_Fromm (accessed August 2018)

F

Faulkner, Steve, et al., "The Effect of Passive Heating on Heat Shock Protein 70 and Interleukin-6: A Possible Treatment Tool for Metabolic Diseases?," *Temperature*, 4/3 (2017), pp. 292–304, www.ncbi.nlm.nih.gov/pubmed/28944271

Fleischner, Thomas Lowe, ed., *Nature, Love, Medicine: Essays on Wildness and Wellness* (Torrey House Press, 2017)

Frank, Matt, "The Human Health and Social Benefits of Urban Forests," Dovetail Partners, September 19, 2016, www.dovetailinc.org/reports/The+Human+Health+and+Social+Benefits+of+Urban+Forests_n782

Fromm, Erich, *The Anatomy of Human Destructiveness* (H. Holt, 1992)

"Functions of the Autonomic Nervous System," Lumen, https://courses.lumenlearning.com/boundless-ap/chapter/functions-of-the-autonomic-nervous-system (accessed August 2018)

Funk, Rainer, *Erich Fromm: His Life and Ideas*, trans. Ian Portman and Manuela Kunkel (Continuum International Publishing Group, 2003)

G

Gander, Kashmira, "Can You Get a Suntan and Absorb Vitamin D through a Window?," *The Independent*, February 25, 2016, www.independent.co.uk/life-style/health-and-families/features/can-you-get-a-tan-and-absorb-vitamin-d-through-a-window-a6895626.html

Gelter, Hans, "*Friluftsliv*: The Scandinavian Philosophy of Outdoor Life," *Canadian Journal of Environmental Education*, 5 (Summer 2000), pp. 77–90, www.natureandforesttherapy.org/uploads/8/1/4/4/8144400/friluftsliv_scandanavian_philosophy_of_outdoor_life.pdf

"Getting Sprung: The Biological Underpinnings of Spring Fever," LabSpaces, June 3, 2013, www.labspaces.net/blog/1621/Getting_Sprung__The_Biological_Underpinnings_of_Spring_Fever

Giaimo, Cara, "The Man Who Recorded, Tamed, and Then Sold Nature Sounds to America," *Atlas Obscura*, April 5, 2016, www.atlasobscura.com/articles/the-man-who-recorded-tamed-and-then-sold-nature-sounds-to-america

Gonzalez, Marianne Thorsen, *Therapeutic Horticulture for Clinical Depression in a Green Care Context (Terapeutisk Hagebruk ved Klinisk Depresjon i en Grønn Omsorg Kontekst)* (Norwegian University of Life Sciences, Department of Plant and Environmental Sciences, 2010)

Gozuyesil, Ebru, and Mürüvvet Baser, "The Effect of Foot Reflexology Applied to Women Aged Between 40 and 60 on Vasomotor Complaints and Quality of Life," *Complementary Therapies in Clinical Practice*, 24 (August 2016), pp. 78–85, www.ncbi.nlm.nih.gov/pubmed/27502805

Green, Peter, *Kenneth Grahame, 1859–1932: A Study of His Life, Work, and Times* (John Murray, 1959)

Groh, Jennifer M., *Making Space, How the Brain Knows Where Things Are* (Belknap Press, 2014)

Gross, Daniel A., "This Is Your Brain on Silence," *Nautilus*, July 7, 2016, www.nautil.us/issue/38/noise/this-is-your-brain-on-silence-rp

Grygny, J.P., "Dancing With Trees, Interviewing Flowers: The Performance Ecology Project," Center for Humans & Nature, March 27, 2018, www.humansandnature.org/dancing-with-trees-interviewing-flowers-the-performance-ecology-project

H

Hamblin, James, "Don't Be Surprised if Your Doctor Prescribes a Park: Why Some Doctors Are Writing Prescriptions for Time Outdoors," *The Atlantic*, September 15, 2015, www.theatlantic.com/magazine/archive/2015/10/the-nature-cure/403210

Hanh, Thich Nhat, *Present Moment, Wonderful Moment* (Parallax Press, 2002)

—, "Thich Nhat Hanh on Walking Meditation," *Lion's Roar*, April 5, 2018, www.lionsroar.com/how-to-meditate-thich-nhat-hanh-on-walking-meditation

Hanson, Rick, *Hardwiring Happiness* (Harmony Books, 2016)

Harvard Health Publishing, "A Prescription for Better Health: Go Alfresco," Harvard Health Letter, July 2010, www.health.harvard.edu/newsletter_article/a-prescription-for-better-health-go-alfresco

Haskell, David G., *The Songs of Trees* (Viking Press, 2017)

Hazen, Teresia, "Therapeutic Garden Characteristics," *Quarterly Publication of the American Horticultural Therapy Association*, 41/2 (2003), https://ahta.memberclicks.net/assets/docs/therapeuticgardencharacteristics_ahtareprintpermission.pdf

Heiser, Christina, "How the Simple Act of Nature Helps You De-stress," *Better*, September 29, 2017, www.nbcnews.com/better/pop-culture/how-nature-can-solve-life-s-most-challenging-problems-ncna749361

Heritage Council, "Children and the Outdoors," 2016, www.heritagecouncil.ie/content/files/children_%20outdoors_commissioned_report_26mb.pdf

Hirschi, Jane S., *Ripe for Change* (Harvard Education Press, 2015)

Hopper, Leigh, "Researchers Link Sedentary Behavior to Thinning in Brain Region Critical for Memory," UCLA Newsroom, April 16,

2018, www.newsroom.ucla.edu/releases/researchers-link-sedentary-behavior-to-thinning-in-brain-region-critical-for-memory

"How to Feel Happy Just By Walking Differently," *PsyBlog*, October 16, 2016, www.spring.org.uk/2014/10/how-to-feel-happy-just-by-walking-differently.ph

I

Ivens, Sarah, "'Forest Bathing' Makes Sense (Even if the Name Might Be Daft)," *The Telegraph*, April 9, 2018, www.telegraph.co.uk/women/life/forest-bathing-makes-sense-even-name-might-daft

J

Jabr, Ferris, "Why Walking Helps Us Think," *New Yorker*, September 3, 2014, www.newyorker.com/tech/elements/walking-helps-us-think

Jaffe, Ali, "Hiking Kumano Kodo, a Remote Ancient Pilgrimage Route in Japan," *Atlas Obscura*, February 6, 2018, www.atlasobscura.com/articles/kumano-kodo

Jarrett, Christian, "Your Brain Performs Better When It's Cold Outside," *CNN*, February 19, 2016, www.cnn.com/2016/02/19/health/your-brain-on-winter/index.html

Jones, Josh, "How Walking Fosters Creativity: Stanford Researchers Confirm What Philosophers and Writers Have Always Known," *Open Culture*, July 8, 2015, www.openculture.com/2015/07/how-walking-fosters-creativity.html

——, "New Study: Immersing Yourself in Art, Music and Nature Might Reduce Inflammation and Increase Life Expectancy," *Open Culture*, August 7, 2015, www.openculture.com/2015/08/new-study-immersing-yourself-in-art-music-nature-might-reduce-inflammation-increase-life-expectancy.html

K

Kaplan, Matt, *Science of the Magical* (Scribner, 2016)

Kardan, Omid, et al., "Neighborhood Greenspace and Health in a Large Urban Center," *Scientific Reports*, 5/1 (2015), www.nature.com/articles/srep11610

Kelmenson, Kalia, "The Potent Power of the Sun," *Spirituality & Health*, June 6, 2017, www.spiritualityhealth.com/blogs/the-present-moment/2017/06/06/kalia-kelmenson-potent-power-sun

Keltner, Dacher, and J. Haidt, "Approaching Awe, a Moral, Spiritual, and Aesthetic Emotion," *Cognition and Emotion*, 17/2 (March 2003), pp. 297–314, www.ncbi.nlm.nih.gov/pubmed/29715721

Khazan, Olga, "How Walking in Nature Prevents Depression," *The Atlantic*, June 30, 2015, www.theatlantic.com/health/archive/2015/06/how-walking-in-nature-prevents-depression/397172

Kimmerer, Robin Wall, *Braiding Sweetgrass* (Milkweed Editions, 2014)

Kingdom, Frederick A.A., "Color Brings Relief to Human Vision," *Nature Neuroscience*, 6/6 (2003), pp. 641–44, www.nature.com/articles/nn1060

Kortge, Carolyn Scott, *Healing Walks for Hard Times* (Trumpeter, 2010)

Kremins, Deborah, "Mountain Wisdom Part I: Earth Connection/Center of Insight," *Spirituality & Health*, March 20, 2018, www.spiritualityhealth.com/articles/2018/03/20/mountain-wisdom-part-i-earth-connection-center-of-insight

Kuo, Ming, "How Might Contact with Nature Promote Human Health? Promising Mechanisms and a Possible Central Pathway," *Frontiers in Psychology*, 6 (2015), p. 1093, www.ncbi.nlm.nih.gov/pmc/articles/PMC4548093/

Kyoto University, "New Gears in Your Sleep Clock: 'Jekyll and Hyde'-like Control System for Sleep," *Science Daily*, July 11, 2018, www.sciencedaily.com/releases/2018/07/180711093205.htm

L

Laird, Shelby Gull, "Hug a Tree: The Evidence Shows It Really Will Make You Feel Better," *The Conversation*, March 18, 2014, www.theconversation.com/hug-a-tree-the-evidence-shows-it-really-will-make-you-feel-better-21924

Lambert, G.W., et al., "Effect of Sunlight and Season on Serotonin Turnover in the Brain," *The Lancet*, 360/9348 (December 7, 2002), pp. 1840–42, www.thelancet.com/pdfs/journals/lancet/PIIS0140673602117375.pdf

Larson, Samantha, "Sound Check: The Quietest Place in the U.S.," *Crosscut*, March 30, 2016, http://features.crosscut.com/sound-check-the-quietest-place-in-the-us

Laskow, Sarah, "Shedding New Light on the Mysteries of Antarctica's Long, Dark Winter," *Atlas Obscura*, May 15, 2018, www.atlasobscura.com/articles/when-is-winter-in-antarctica

Lawton, Rebecca, "The Healing Power of Nature," *Aeon*, September 6, 2017, www.aeon.co/essays/why-forests-and-rivers-are-the-most-potent-health-tonic-around

Lee, Helena, "The Babies Who Nap in Sub-zero Temperatures," *BBC News*, February 22, 2013, www.bbc.com/news/magazine-21537988

Lewis, Tim, "Meet the Man Living with Alzheimer's Who Climbs the Same Mountain Every Day," *The Guardian*, March 25, 2018, www.theguardian.com/lifeandstyle/2018/mar/25/meet-the-man-living-with-alzheimers-who-climbs-the-same-mountain-every-day

Li, Qing, *Forest Bathing* (Penguin, 2018)

——, "'Forest Bathing' Is Great for Your Health. Here's How to Do It," *Time*, May 1, 2018, www.time.com/5259602/japanese-forest-bathing

Louv, Richard, *Last Child in the Woods* (Algonquin Books, 2005)

——, *Vitamin N* (Atlantic Books, 2017)

M

Maffit, Rev. John Newland, *Calvary Token, and Literary Souvenir* (1846), available at https://play.google.com/books/reader?id=7mQiAQAAMAAJ

"Make Your Sit Spot Practice Private and Intimate," *In My Nature*, January 25, 2017, www.inmynature.life/make-sit-spot-practice-private-intimate

Malchik, Antonia, "Follow Your Feet," *Orion Magazine*, www.orionmagazine.org/article/follow-your-feet (accessed August 2018)

Martinko, Katherine, "Children Spend Less Time Outside than Prison Inmates," *TreeHugger*, February 5, 2018, www.treehugger.com/culture/children-spend-less-time-outside-prison-inmates.html

McLuhan, T.C., *The Way of the Earth* (Simon & Schuster, 1994)

Mills, Billy, "Path to Enlightenment: How Walking Inspires Writers," *The Guardian*, August 9, 2012, www.theguardian.com/books/2012/aug/09/how-walking-inspires-writers

Miss Mollett, "The Nurse and the Sick-Room," *The Hospital*, 2/41 (1887), pp. 245–46

Morris, Roderick Conway, "Early Slices of Paradise: Gardens in Ancient Times," *New York Times*, July 13, 2007, www.nytimes.com/2007/07/12/arts/12iht-conway.1.6629841.html

Mowe, Sam, "A Garden for Enlightenment: An Interview with Martin Mosko," *Spirituality & Health*, April 24, 2018, www.spiritualityhealth.com/articles/2018/04/24/a-garden-for-enlightenment

N

Navarrete, David, and Bill Witherspoon, "Mind over Matter: The Restorative Impact of Perceived Open Space," *Conscious Cities*, June 4, 2018, www.ccities.org/mind-matter-restorative-impact-perceived-open-space

Neale, Miles, *Gradual Awakening* (Sounds True, 2018)

Neimark, Jill, "The Camping Cure," *Aeon*, January 22, 2014, www.aeon.co/essays/environmental-illness-made-me-too-sick-to-live-inside

Nichols, Wallace J., *Blue Mind* (Little, Brown, 2014)

Nietzsche, Friedrich Wilhelm, Keith Ansell-Pearson, and Duncan Large, *The Nietzsche Reader* (Blackwell Publishing, 2006)

Nightingale, Florence, *Notes on Nursing and Notes on Hospitals* (Classics of Medicine Library, 1982)

Niteshad, "Grounding: Healing Practices," *Shamans Cave*, www.shamanscave.com/practices/grounding (accessed August 2018)

O

O'Connor, Joanne, "Trees of Life: Forest Bathing Blossoms in Britain," *The Guardian*, May 6, 2018, www.theguardian.com/travel/2018/may/06/japanese-art-of-forest-bathing-comes-to-england-holidays

Office for National Statistics, "Children's Engagement with the Outdoors and Sports Activities, UK: 2014 to 2015," 2018, www.ons.gov.uk/peoplepopulationandcommunity/wellbeing/articles/childrensengagementwiththeoutdoorsandsportsactivitiesuk/2014to2015

P

Park, Shin-Jung, and Hiromi Tokura, "Bright Light Exposure During the Daytime Affects Circadian Rhythms of Urinary Melatonin and Salivary Immunoglobulin A," *Chronobiology International*, 16/3 (May 16, 1999), pp. 359–71, www.ncbi.nlm.nih.gov/pubmed/10373104

Parramore, Lynn, "The Average American Worker Takes Less Vacation Time than a Medieval Peasant," *Business Insider*, November 7, 2016, www.businessinsider.com/american-worker-less-vacation-medieval-peasant-2016-11

"Perceiving the Light," European Lighting School, www.lightingschool.eu/portfolio/1-perceiving-the-light (accessed August 2018)

Physiological Society, "Effects of Night-time Light on Internal Body Clock," *Science Daily*, April 30, 2018, www.sciencedaily.com/releases/2018/04/180430075635.htm

Popova, Maria, "Ode to a Flower: Richard Feynman's Famous Monologue on Knowledge and Mystery, Animated," *Brain Pickings*, January 3, 2018, www.brainpickings.org/2013/01/01/ode-to-a-flower-richard-feynman

—, "Walking as Creative Fuel: A Splendid 1913 Celebration of How Solitary Walks Enliven 'The Country of the Mind,'" *Brain Pickings*, January 22, 2018, www.brainpickings.org/2018/01/10/kenneth-grahame-the-fellow-that-goes-alone

Press Association, "Children Spend Only Half as Much Time Playing Outside as Their Parents Did," *The Guardian*, July 27, 2016, www.theguardian.com/environment/2016/jul/27/children-spend-only-half-the-time-playing-outside-as-their-parents-did

R

Ratcliffe, Eleanor, *Restorative Perceptions and Outcomes Associated with Listening to Birds*, PhD diss., University of Surrey, 2015, http://epubs.surrey.ac.uk/808249

Ryan, Richard M., et al., "Vitalizing Effects of Being Outdoors and in Nature," *Journal of Environmental Psychology*, 30/2 (2010), pp. 159–68, www.sciencedirect.com/science/article/pii/S0272494409000838

S

Saeki, Yuka, "The Effect of Foot-bath With or Without the Essential Oil of Lavender on the Autonomic Nervous System: A Randomized Trial," *Complementary Therapies in Medicine*, 8/1 (2000), pp. 2–7, www.ncbi.nlm.nih.gov/pubmed/10812753

Satish, Usha, et al., "Is CO_2 an Indoor Pollutant? Direct Effects of Low-to-Moderate CO_2 Concentrations on Human Decision-Making Performance," *Environmental Health Perspectives*, 120/12 (December 2012), pp. 1671–77, www.ncbi.nlm.nih.gov/pmc/articles/PMC3548274/

Schlanger, Zoë, "Dirt Has a Microbiome, and It May Double as an Antidepressant," *Quartz*, May 30, 2017, www.qz.com/993258/dirt-has-a-microbiome-and-it-may-double-as-an-antidepressant

Schor, Juliet B., *The Overworked American* (BasicBooks, 1993)

Schreiber, Melody, "Solving the Suicide Crisis in the Arctic Circle," *Pacific Standard*, March 23, 2018, www.psmag.com/environment/solving-the-suicide-crisis-in-the-arctic-circle

Selhub, Eva M., and Alan C. Logan, *Your Brain On Nature* (John Wiley & Sons, 2012)

Shanahan, Mike, *Gods, Wasps and Stranglers: The Secret History and Redemptive Future of Fig Trees* (Chelsea Green, 2018)

—, "Why Forests Give You Awe: Facts so Romantic," *Nautilus*, March 21, 2018, www.nautil.us/blog/why-forests-give-you-awe

Siddarth, Prabha, et al., "Sedentary Behavior Associated with Reduced Medial Temporal Lobe Thickness in Middle-aged and

Older Adults," *PLoS One*, 13/4 (April 2018), www.journals.plos.org/plosone/article?id=10.1371/journal.pone.0195549

Snyder, Gary, *The Practice of the Wild* (Counterpoint, 1990)

Snyder, Kimberly, "Why Going Barefoot Is Actually Good for You," *Well+Good*, April 2, 2018, www.wellandgood.com/good-advice/what-is-grounding-kimberly-snyder

Starks, Philip T.B., "Would You Like a Side of Dirt with That?," *Scientific American*, June 1, 2012, www.scientificamerican.com/article/would-you-like-side-dirt-eating-soil

Sternberg, Esther M., *Healing Spaces* (Belknap Press, 2010)

Strand, Clark, *Waking Up to the Dark* (Spiegel & Grau, 2015)

Suttie, Jill, "How Nature Can Make You Kinder, Happier, and More Creative," *Greater Good*, March 2, 2016, www.greatergood.berkeley.edu/article/item/how_nature_makes_you_kinder_happier_more_creative

T

Texas A&M University, "Breast Cancer Linked to the Body's Internal Clock," *Science Daily*, May 8, 2018, www.sciencedaily.com/releases/2018/05/180508170901.htm

Tilley, Sara, et al., "Older People's Experiences of Mobility and Mood in an Urban Environment: A Mixed Methods Approach Using Electroencephalography (EEG) and Interviews," *International Journal of Environmental Research and Public Health*, 14/2 (2017), p. 151, www.ncbi.nlm.nih.gov/pubmed/28165409

Toomey, Diane, "How Listening to Trees Can Help Reveal Nature's Connections," *Yale Environment 360*, August 24, 2017, www.e360.yale.edu/features/how-listening-to-trees-can-help-reveal-natures-connections

Tuhus-Dubrow, Rebecca, "What a Park's Design Does to Your Brain," *Next City*, September 23, 2014, www.nextcity.org/daily/entry/city-parks-design-calming-brain

Tzelnic, Alex, "Can Nature Experiences Replace Mindfulness?," Garrison Institute blog, June 2, 2018, www.garrisoninstitute.org/blog/nature-and-mindfulness

U

University of East Anglia, "It's Official—Spending Time Outside Is Good for You," *Science Daily*, July 6, 2018, www.sciencedaily.com/releases/2018/07/180706102842.htm

University of Kent, "Why We Struggle to Get Good Night's Sleep as We Get Older," *Science Daily*, March 27, 2018, www.sciencedaily.com/releases/2018/03/180327102829.htm

University of Michigan, "Get Moving to Get Happier, Study Finds," *Science Daily*, April 4, 2018, www.sciencedaily.com/releases/2018/04/180404163635.htm

University of Seville, "Human Daily Rhythms: Clocks vs Light/Dark Cycle," *Science Daily*, April 3, 2018, www.sciencedaily.com/releases/2018/04/180403090052.htm

University of Twente, "Worldwide Degradation of Land and Nature Threatens Prosperity and Wellbeing," *Science Daily*, March 27, 2018, www.sciencedaily.com/releases/2018/03/180327111611.htm

"U.S. Study Shows Widening Disconnect with Nature, and Potential Solutions," *Yale Environment 360*, April 27, 2017, www.e360.yale.edu/digest/u-s-study-shows-widening-disconnect-with-nature-and-potential-solutions

USDA Forest Service—Northern Research Station, "Growing Need for Urban Forests as Urban Land Expands," *Science Daily*, March 14, 2018, www.sciencedaily.com/releases/2018/03/180314101954.htm

V

Veder, Robin, "Mother-Love for Plant-Children: Sentimental Pastoralism and Nineteenth-Century Parlour Gardening," *Australasian Journal of American Studies*, 26/2 (2007), pp. 20–34, www.jstor.org/stable/41054074

von Lindern, E., F. Lymeus, and T. Hartig, "The Restorative Environment: A Complementary Concept for Salutogenesis Studies," in *The Handbook of Salutogenesis*, ed. M.B. Mittelmark et al. (Springer; 2017)

W

Wade, Betsy, "There's Nothing Dainty About a Mud Bath," *New York Times*, December 8, 1996, www.nytimes.com/1996/12/08/travel/there-s-nothing-dainty-about-a-mud-bath.html

Walljasper, Jay, "The Positive Power of Walking," *Utne Reader*, June 27, 2017, www.utne.com/mind-and-body/the-positive-power-of-walking-zbtz1706zsau

"Watching Nature Programmes Makes You Happier New Research Reveals," BBC Media Centre, March 8, 2017, www.bbc.co.uk/mediacentre/worldwide/2017/rhp

Weil, Elizabeth, "The Woman Who Walked 10,000 Miles (No Exaggeration) in Three Years," *New York Times*, September 25, 2014, www.nytimes.com/2014/09/28/magazine/the-woman-who-walked-10000-miles-no-exaggeration-in-three-years.html

Whittaker, Richard, "An Interview with Betsy Damon: Living Water," December 25, 2009, www.conversations.org/story.php?sid=222

Williams, Conor, "The Perks of a Play-in-the-Mud Educational Philosophy," *The Atlantic*, April 27, 2018, www.theatlantic.com/education/archive/2018/04/early-childhood-outdoor-education/558959

Williams, Florence, "The Adventure Therapy Cure for Survivors," *Outside*, May 1, 2018, www.outsideonline.com/2291381/survivors

—, *The Nature Fix* (W.W. Norton & Company, 2017)

—, "This Is Your Brain on Nature," *National Geographic*, July 25, 2017, www.nationalgeographic.com/magazine/2016/01/call-to-wild

Wilson, Edward Osborne, *Biophilia* (Harvard University Press, 1984)

Wise, Abigail, "Why Getting Fresh Air Is So Good for You," *Huffington Post*, December 6, 2017, www.huffingtonpost.com/2014/08/08/tk-ways-fresh-air-impacts_0_n_5648164.html

Wohlleben, Peter, *Hidden Life of Trees* (HarperCollins Publishers, 2017)

—, *The Weather Detective* (Rider, 2018)

INDEX

CREDITS

pp. 31, 119, and 120: *Waking Up to the Dark* by Clark Strand (Spiegel & Grau, 2015).

p. 108: "Water Meditation" from "Sacred Water" by Bonnie Myotai Treace (2016) reprinted with permission of the author.

p. 108: "Water Meditation" adapted from *Gradual Awakening: The Tibetan Buddhist Path of Becoming Fully Human*, by Miles Neale PsyD, copyright 2018, Boulder, Colorado: Sounds True. Reprinted and adapted with permission of the author.

p. 130: "Sky Gazing" from *Make Me One with Everything: Buddhist Meditations to Awaken from the Illusion of Separation* by Lama Surya Das, founder of the Dzogchen Center, Dzogchen Retreats, copyright 2015, Boulder, Colorado: Sounds True. Reprinted and adapted with permission of the author.

Photography

Key: b = below, a = above, l = left, c = center, r = right, bkg = background

© RYLAND PETERS AND SMALL/CICO BOOKS

Caroline Arber: p. 105.
Jan Baldwin: pp. 20 (a house in Cape Elizabeth designed by Stephen Blatt Architects), 101.
Simon Brown: p. 79.
Earl Carter: pp. 9, 21 (bkg), 121 (bkg), 130 (bkg).
Helen Cathcart: pp. 4, 49, 125, 126.
Peter Cassidy: pp. 85, 115.
Amanda Darcy: p. 17.
Christopher Drake: p. 21 (Florence and Pierre Pallardy, Domaine de la Baronnie, Saint-Martin de Ré).

Dylan Drummond: p. 44 (bkg).
Dan Duchars: pp. 104, 112.
Chris Everard: p. 31.
Erika Flores: pp. 92–95 (taken from *The Yoga Healer* by Christine Burke).
Georgia Glynn-Smith: pp. 41 (bkg), 42, 65b.
Caroline Hughes: pp. 51, 61, 65a, 65c.
Kim Lightbody: p. 87.
Mark Lohman: p. 120.
David Merewether: pp. 71, 118, 129; also bkgs pp. 4–5, 32–33, 66–67, 80–81.
Emma Mitchell: pp. 5, 67.
Peter Moore: pp. 7, 24, 80, 102.

Andrew Wood: p. 13.
Polly Wreford: pp. 14 (Ingrid and Avinash Persaud's home in London), 33.
Steve Painter: pp. 2, 27, 39.
Debbie Patterson: p. 73a.
Claire Richardson: pp. 19c, 19r.
Mark Scott: pp. 92–95 (bkg).
Lucinda Symons: pp. 3, 40, 76, 81.
Debi Treloar: pp. 19l, 28, 32, 63, 90, 117 (www.helenbraby. co.uk), 121 (the guesthouse of the interior designer & artist Philippe Guilmin, Brussels).
Chris Tubbs: pp. 36, 74 (bkg), 91, 98, 107, 108–109 (bkg).
Ian Wallace: p. 72.
Stuart West: p. 75.
Kate Whitaker: p. 99.

SHUTTERSTOCK
© Riccardo Arata: p. 52.
© barmalini: p. 55.
© Martin Castrogiovanni: p. 109.
© Humannet: p. 88 (bkg).
© Young Swee Ming: p. 73b.

Edina van der Wyck: p. 43.
Francesca Yorke: p. 59.

ACKNOWLEDGMENTS

Thank you to the patient and wise team at CICO Books—Carmel Edmonds, Cindy Richards, Kristine Pidkameny, Emily Breen, and Rosie Fairhead. Thanks as well to Katherine Snelson, Dr. Pooja Amy Shah, and my agent Susan Lee Cohen who helped form and finesse the ideas for this book. I'm grateful to Lama Surya Das, Miles Neale, and Bonnie Myotai Treace for the gift of their teachings, and to Duane Stapp who is always my best first reader.